Affective Teaching in Nursing

Dennis Ondrejka, PhD, RN, CNS, is currently the director of nursing programs and professor at Colorado Christian University in Northglenn, Colorado. Dr. Ondrejka has worked to build a Shared Governance Program moving toward Magnet recognition for Exempla Lutheran Medical Center in Wheat Ridge, Colorado, just prior to returning to education. He is an advanced practice nurse in Colorado in the specialty of community and occupational health and received his master's in nursing from the University of Wisconsin, Milwaukee in 1981. As a specialist in occupational health, he worked as a clinician and manager for several nationally acclaimed agencies, such as the National Jewish Hospital in Denver, Children's Hospital in Denver, General Motors (AC Spark Plug Division) in Oak Creek, Wisconsin, and Manville Corporation in Denver.

Dr. Ondrejka received his doctorate at the University of Denver in higher education in 1998 with a dissertation focused on "Affective Pedagogy in Post-Baccalaureate Education." He began his teaching career in 1982 at the University of Wisconsin, Milwaukee, where his expertise was mental health and addiction detoxification. Since receiving his doctorate, Dr. Ondrejka taught at the University of Utah-College of Nursing and at Regis University before becoming an associate professor and associate dean at the Denver School of Nursing.

Dr. Ondrejka has presented and published on numerous topics, including emotional intelligence in nursing, relationship-based care strategies, unstructured problem solving, occupational health specialty topics, and the patient experience in health care. This is Dr. Ondrejka's first book focused on his passion, teaching in the affective domain for nursing students.

Affective Teaching in Nursing

Connecting to Feelings, Values, and Inner Awareness

Dennis Ondrejka, PhD, RN, CNS

Springer Publishing Company, LLC
11 West 42nd Street
New York, NY 10036
www.springerpub.com

Acquisitions Editor: Margaret Zuccarini
Composition: AMNET

ISBN: 978-0-8261-1792-2
e-book ISBN: 978-0-8261-1793-9

13 14 15 16 17 / 5 4 3 2 1

Library of Congress Cataloging-in-Publication Data

Ondrejka, Dennis.
Affective teaching in nursing : connecting to feelings, values, and inner awareness / Dennis Ondrejka.
p. ; cm.
Includes bibliographical references and index.
ISBN 978-0-8261-1792-2 (print edition : alk. paper) – ISBN 978-0-8261-1793-9 (e-book)
I. Title.
[DNLM: 1. Education, Nursing–methods. 2. Philosophy, Nursing. 3. Teaching–methods. WY 18]
RT84.5
610.7301–dc23

2013013667

Printed in the United States of America by Gasch Printing.

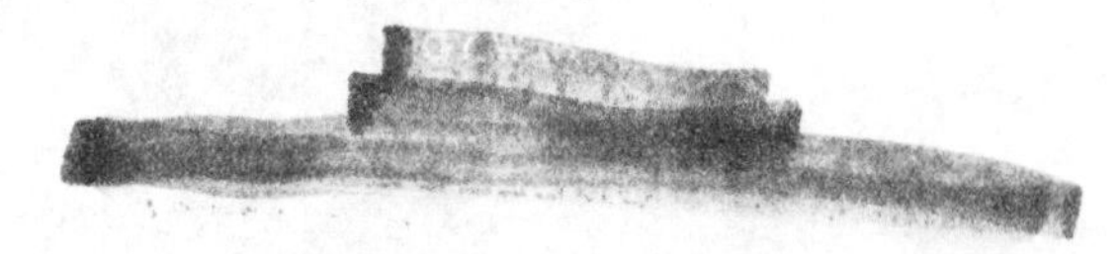

My educational path has had many mentors and guides, but none as supportive and guiding as Dr. Jim Davis, who was my professor and dissertation chair as I built my thinking regarding the topic of affective pedagogy. I dedicate this book to him as a thank you for his dedication to me, and higher education in general, at the University of Denver and the University of Denver College.

Contents

PART III: INTEGRATING AFFECTIVE TEACHING IN NURSING: THE BIG PICTURE IN NURSING EDUCATION

Foreword

In 1909 Richard Olding Beard, the founder of the School of Nursing at the University of Minnesota, wrote an article titled, "The Educated Spirit of the Nurse." In it he says, "The educated spirit of the nurse can thrive and grow and find its ultimate satisfaction and fulfillment only in the fact that it serves, and that its service is inspired by love." Dr. Beard sees the profession of nursing as one without boundaries—one that is limitless in reaching for the health of society. Dennis Ondrejka's book, *Affective Teaching in Nursing,* is about building a curriculum for nurse educators to teach future nurses how to reach a goal of whole-person involvement in the service of creating a healthy society.

The goal of whole-person involvement was first brought to me many years ago in an article by Sister Madeleine Clemence. It was published in 1966 in the *American Journal of Nursing,* and it was called "Existentialism: A Philosophy of Commitment." Even that long ago, she was challenging people to bring their whole selves to their work:

> Commitment can mean many things: a promise to keep, a sense of dedication that transcends all other considerations, an unswerving allegiance to a given point of view. In existentialism, commitment means even more: a willingness to live fully one's own life, to make that life meaningful through acceptance of, rather than detachment from, all that it may hold of both joy and sorrow.

It is important to note that she was talking specifically about a nurse's work when she spoke of the absolute essentialness of, "acceptance of, rather than detachment from, all that life may hold." While observing herself and her nurse peers, Sister Madeleine could see that the work of the nurse is secular for all, but sacred for only those who commit themselves to making it sacred.

But that was long ago. What is the world of the nurse like now?

Do we as nurses invite ourselves into the mystery of what it means to be with a person who is suffering, vulnerable, and afraid? Do we allow ourselves to be involved with our patients? This is challenging language, as we have been warned against *over*-involvement for as long as there have been nurses. But are we now living out a tragically over-corrected version of that perfectly reasonable caveat? If I am not involved with my patients, can they possibly feel as though I'll be there for them when they need me?

Ondrejka understands the necessity of infusing today's fast-paced, technically challenging, often chaotic care environments with the absolute imperative that we bring our whole selves to our work. There is no doubt that it's hard. There are obstacles to nurses bringing their whole selves to their work with patients today, and there will be a whole new set of obstacles tomorrow. It's possible, though, and anything less than whole-person engagement in our work is not sustainable.

In this book, Ondrejka connects many dots for me in the creation of a curriculum for nurse educators to teach future nurses how to reach a goal of whole-person involvement. First of all, he connects the dots of affective teaching in nursing with the concept of relationship-based care, which, to me, exemplifies the nursing imperative.

The way I see it, the nursing imperative is a two-sided coin. On one side there is the imperative to be clinically competent in both technical skills and clinical judgment. The other side is the willingness to step into *being with* the human being for whom the nurse is caring. In health care, people experience vulnerability at every level of their being: mental, emotional, physical, and spiritual. The privilege of nursing is having the knowledge and skill, the position and relationship, to interact with a vulnerable human being in a way that alleviates pain and increases mental, emotional, physical, and spiritual comfort. This is the privilege of nursing—the *being with* a vulnerable human being. And if this privilege is ignored or overlooked, nursing isn't happening. Just doing tasks is not nursing; it is just doing tasks. No matter what is happening in a care environment, authentic human connection with the vulnerable human beings in our care can and must happen.

I believe that all nursing students who are fortunate enough to have this book as a text will be given an extraordinary opportunity that I hope will one day become common place. As I write this, I am heartened to know that conversations will be taking place in classrooms across the world about the value of therapeutic relationships—about the wisdom of becoming professionally involved with patients and families, about the gifts those relationships give, and about the ways in which authentic relationships with patients and families will sustain caregivers, preventing burnout and compassion fatigue. I have seen again and again that caregivers get energy from human connection. Without this energy, compassion is not sustainable.

To know oneself is an important skill in being able to create a therapeutic relationship. There are many resources that can help in this endeavor—most notably the work that Dr. Brené Brown is doing on vulnerability as the seat of creativity, and the work that Mary Koloroutis and Michael Trout have documented in their book, *See Me as a Person: Creating Therapeutic Relationships*

with Patients and their Families. Clearly the vital work of educating nurses holistically—mind, body, and spirit—is gaining traction.

Holistic nursing is the wave of the future, and affective education is a sturdy ladder to be climbed by educators in order to develop nurses with "educated spirits." And let's take one more look at exactly what the venerable Richard Olding Beard meant by that: "The educated spirit of the nurse can thrive and grow and find its ultimate satisfaction and fulfillment only in the fact that it serves, and that its service is inspired by love."

It doesn't get any more personal than that.

I am both honored and humbled to be in a position to encourage you to read this book carefully and to take it to heart.

Marie Manthey, MNA, FRCN, FAAN
Founder, Creative Health Care Management

REFERENCE

Clemence, M. (1966). Existentialism: A philosophy of commitment. *American Journal of Nursing, 66*(3), 500–505.

Preface

WHY THIS? WHY NOW?

Ask yourself if you have become accustomed to and dependent on the traditional models of education, or are you ready to explore something else? If you want something different that will impact students' values, feelings, and inner awareness—then this is the right place and this text is for you. In *Affective Teaching in Nursing: Connecting to Feelings, Values, and Inner Awareness,* the reader should face up to what is the norm in nursing education when only a small portion of the whole student is taught. Many now realize that nursing education today has not progressed as anticipated through the 21st century, leaving the affective domain of education absent in most settings. This text contributes new ideas that have not surfaced in most nursing classrooms and reinforces old ideas. It provides the reader with additional insights into why affective methods have not been practiced. In addition, this text will assist nursing educators who are motivated toward affective teaching methods to find the necessary tools and to understand the challenge facing affective educators.

> ... I was formed—or
> deformed—in the educational
> systems of this country
> to live out of the top inch
> and half of the human self;
> to live exclusively through
> cognitive rationality and the
> powers of the intellect; to live
> out of touch with anything
> that lay below that top inch
> and half—body, intuition,
> feeling, emotion, relationship.
> (Palmer,1999, p. 17)

The topic of changing the way educators teach has historical and current relevance in nursing education. Educators often state there is a need for balance between affective and cognitive teaching methods. However, they have difficulty knowing how such pedagogy is possible. *Affective Teaching in Nursing* examines the shifting academic thought and the historical loss or failure to begin affective teaching, tracing it from the 1960s to the present.

During this period, various academic programs have seen a resurgence in what might be considered affective pedagogy with the integration of social and emotional learning and significant philosophical shifts in what it means to educate the whole student. This resurgence was less visible in higher education settings, which has led to growing frustration for those who have desired to see variations of affective pedagogy being sustained in nursing settings, especially in the 1970s with the work of Jean Watson.

> Attitudes, feelings, goals, values, beliefs, and the past experiences influence behavior. When I feel good about myself and my situation, I act in the manner that reflects my positive attitude; conversely, when I feel cynical or depressed or just tired, that attitude is reflected in my behavior. Everything I do, whether it's the way I walk or the way I respond to a student's glance, is intimately related to how I see myself and my environment. . . . (Curwin & Fuhrman, 1975, p. 19)

In the past 10 to 15 years we saw the affective trend shaping itself. This has brought a host of educators together as they evaluate, conduct research, and explore the affective domain of teaching. Nursing was a critical part of that movement and we found ourselves wondering what it means to be teaching in the affective domain. Affective teaching has either been a mystery of meaning or at the very least confusing for educators to bring into their practices. Imagine having the teaching tools that would promote the growth of nursing students' subjective selves, values, beliefs, feelings, and relational and inner awareness. Nurses need this level of self-awareness to be truly connected to their patients during the healing process, as well as to understand their therapeutic selves. Affective teaching is at the core of all *care pedagogy*—it is time to know more about what that means.

> Some teachers recognize the flaws of their approach. Commented one, "We can teach in this program, we can teach in that program, and I don't necessarily feel that's true education, when you become so multitask, that you put everything on a PowerPoint and you pull it out of the drawer." Her colleague added, "Homogenized is what I call it." (Benner, Sutphen, Leonard & Day, 2010, p. 67)

The information presented in this text has never been more relevant because now there is a new generation of students who may find nursing education to be a heartless endeavor without soul. In addition, there is a significant exiting process of retiring faculty who likely never made a comprehensive shift away from the traditional teaching methods learned from past education mentors. The point to be made is that traditional nursing students and other adult learners want more than knowledge being tossed in their direction in the hope that some specific information will stick. Students today want to know if the disseminated new knowledge impacts them in a personal way—through affective development. Nursing students want to know if what they are learning can actually nurture their clinical futures and feed their brains, which makes them feel knowledgeable and alive. Then there are those who only want the information given to them so they can check off a course and move on. The challenge in teaching this latter group is to assist them to have a sense of valuing affective education and development. I believe the material in this text is capable of creating a new generation of affectively literate nurses who understand how they fit into a true caring relationship with their patients.

Traditional teaching is teacher-focused pedagogy where instruction is about the instructor's comfort, level of energy, or hidden agenda and not necessarily about learning. It is convenient, easy, and sounds more objective—but at a cost. Now is the time to be more aware of what affective education means and what it would look like in nursing education today.

Affective Teaching in Nursing is an academic text that takes the reader into the world of theory, analysis, practice, and the possibilities of affective pedagogy. The material is referenced and self-reflective for readers to build their toolbox for creating affective literacy in their students if they so choose. It offers the reader a way to assess the classroom and match it to the theoretical premises behind such classroom methods. It is intended to offer something for every type of nursing educator:

- You may be an educator who has been looking for others to join you in your affective teaching strategies—we are here.
- You may be an educator who has been utilizing many powerful classroom strategies, but never knew what to call them—now you will know.
- You may be skeptical and have no intention of integrating this material—maybe you will be convinced to the contrary.

The path laid out within this text is not truly linear in the time frames presented, but the dates give a perspective of various periods that promoted certain themes of affective pedagogy. End and start dates actually overlap. However, it is simply one way to examine shifts in thought on the topic of affective pedagogy in theory and in practice.

The intended audience is nursing educators who are teaching students or those learning to be nursing educators and who need a course in affective teaching. Higher education environments have continuously struggled to put affective education back into curricula from the time Bloom created his affective taxonomy in 1964. It would be valuable for any discipline, but this text is aimed at the foundations of nursing education and speaks of what has not been spoken about effectively over the years.

> Nursing educators are responsible for creating an environment in classroom, laboratory, and clinical settings that facilitates student learning and the achievement of cognitive, *affective*, and psychomotor outcomes. (National League for Nursing, Core Competencies of Nurse Educators, 2005, p. 1 [italics added])

Recent events have increased the need to bring this work forward. The Institute of Medicine (IOM, 2011) report on the future of nursing education asked for several changes, including the need to move away from cognitive memorization.

> New approaches and educational models must be developed to respond to burgeoning information in the field. For example, fundamental concepts that can be applied across all settings and in different situations need to be taught, rather than requiring rote memorization. (p. 2)

Benner, Sutphen, Leonard, and Day (2010) have also been challenging the nursing education system to make radical changes. One of their four recommendations is to move "from an emphasis on socialization and role taking to an emphasis on formation" (p. 89). Their terminology actually goes deeper than a sense of self-awareness—it presents a complex inner sense of *being* rather than *acting* as a nurse. Here is one story they quote from a new nurse who contextualizes the meaning of *becoming a nurse*:

> We are privy to these very, very critical moments in people's lives. Especially, because a lot of us are younger, most of us have never experienced any of these feelings. . . . All of a sudden you are in a room with somebody who's just been told that they may only have a couple of more weeks to live, or that the treatment they're getting isn't working, or that they have the diagnosis that they've been fearing. For us to be there standing by and experiencing that suddenly puts us in a very intimate relation with them. (p. 165)

How are educators to assist their students to attain this level of sensitivity? Are they willing to go to that intimate place in education where tears may be shed? We may be hopeful that these nursing students will personally touch the souls of their patients with their compassion and inner healer, and we need teaching methods that will allow this to happen. The goal of *Affective Teaching in Nursing* is to offer nursing educators ways of achieving these affective goals.

ORGANIZATION

The text is organized into three parts and 12 chapters. The first part is titled "The Problem in Nursing Education." Chapter 1 provides the definition of affective teaching and describes the underlying foundations that start to capture the gifts and risks involved. It provides basic teaching theories that are tied to affective methods, and describes the historical journey of how affective pedagogy was first constructed within Bloom's Taxonomy, and gives some contrast to what it means today. Chapter 1 speaks to the risks for faculty, gives examples of what it has cost faculty to stay true to affective teaching, and demonstrates how others have buffered themselves from such risk.

Chapter 2 presents the definition of traditional teaching and how it works. It encourages the reader to make some historical sense of how we have created a traditional teaching method in nursing that is universal without conscious effort to integrate the affective domain. It includes faculty's use of strategies found to be useful without faculty being able to articulate that many of these are affective pedagogy. The entire process creates a muddy acceptance of what might be accomplished if we were clear about putting affective pedagogy into the curriculum.

Chapter 3 discusses the relationship of affective pedagogy to the subjective world. This chapter considers how the unique and valuable partnership between the two can be researched using qualitative methods and quantum thinking. As educators, we have typically rejected the subjective in favor of being more objective. We now can see that an absence of the subjective has led to a subtle resistance to integrate the affective domain of knowing with a continuous erosion of such teaching methods because of their subjective nature.

Part II, "Affective Concepts, Strategies, and Methods," contains five chapters exploring what we know about affective pedagogy today and how it is being used. Chapter 4 calls out for an infrastructure that can prepare and keep *affective teachers* in nursing. It describes the models that keep such a teaching structure alive and well, avoiding the historical trend that affective educators tend to fade and go away. To encourage affective teaching, this chapter addresses how to prepare yourself as an educator and how to center a group of students. It also examines the role of proxemics (physical environment) in teaching and how to use aesthetics to teach affectively. The chapter closes with building expertise in reflective practices to gain inner awareness.

Chapter 5 explores the philosophical adjustment needed in nursing to move into affective teaching more fully. This chapter suggests several domains in which affective teaching can be used (e.g., aesthetic models and reflection methods). There are philosophical issues within care theory and quantum mechanics that are rarely touched but need to be explored to address the subjective experiences of teaching and learning that result in very different mindsets than what are found in traditional nursing education.

Chapter 6 examines a taxonomy that supports the measuring of what we do in the classroom and therefore promotes the improvement, change, or restructuring of our affective pedagogical methods. This includes the ability to measure the subjective using qualitative methods or even quantum thinking—and this is a challenging thought for some. The chapter's appendix table is an assessment tool that can be used to objectively assess the types of affective teaching methods used in classrooms; this tool was used to collect some of the data found in this text.

Chapter 7 discusses the challenges and achievements of using affective pedagogy in the context of distance learning. There is little research speaking to this directly, but we have been asking educators what they are using to address distance learning. We can extrapolate from other research on the use of distance learning and integrate our understanding of affective methods to look at their value in this form of teaching and to explore the need for additional research for better distance learning practices. Chapter 7 looks at future learning and current challenges posed by academic cheating and how technology supports sophistication in teaching and in cheating.

The last chapter in this part is "Moving From Presentation Slides to Affective Teaching at Conferences." Chapter 8 is for those faculty who have to go to conferences and present their specialty thinking, research, or innovations. Educators are asked to speak at conferences on a regular basis. They are asked to submit their PowerPoints and objectives by a specific date. Not only will many violate the etiquette of doing PowerPoint construction, but many often never move to an interactive presentation model, let alone to the affective domain of learning during any part of a presentation. Chapter 8 encourages the educator to do both.

Part III, "Integrating Affective Teaching in Nursing: The Big Picture in Nursing Education," explores nursing education as an evolving process that went through a maturation phase from the late 1980s to 2003 and included some large academic initiatives in nursing education. Chapter 9 explains why this topic is so important and explores what affective teaching can mean to each educator personally. It continues with a historical perspective on the *care* nursing pedagogy that started to flourish during this period with entire nursing programs using care as a central core of knowing for the student and graduate nurse. The care pedagogy was led by nursing pioneers, including Jean Watson, Madeleine Leininger, D. A. Gaut, Olivia Bevis, and the education pioneer Nel Nodding. It was a time of exploring the idea of care as a unique way of *being* that included skills that needed to be separate from the overall definition of what nurses do with patients. These debates raised the consciousness on nursing theory and continue to this day.

The emotional intelligence movement is presented in Chapter 10 as part of the affective development in education that later merged with the social intelligence movement to be called social–emotional learning (SEL). This movement, seen in the United States and abroad, has significant correlates to affective literacy but has rarely been articulated in nursing programs. However, SEL is demonstrated to be a major focus for other affective educational curricula—especially K–12.

Chapter 11 explores some of the international perspectives found within the SEL movement and its relationship to affective pedagogy emerging in some European and Asian countries. Other nations appear to be attempting to teach to the "whole" student using SEL strategies but without a continuing long-term model.

Chapter 12 encourages us to explore the deeper possibilities, examining why we may have lost something greater than a passion for teaching in the affective. It challenges all of us to identify what may be a serious loss of passion for all teaching; to include our *soul* as teachers and why we may be hiding behind the creation of sterile, cognitive, or heartless classrooms.

This chapter challenges teachers to do their own personal work examining what keeps them separate from others—especially students. Nursing has a history of using *professional distancing* in our clinical practices that has been challenged in more recent years. I believe the same change is needed in the classroom.

There should be learning centers that allow faculty to explore and reclaim their soulful selves. Are you willing to break all the illusions you may have created about yourself and your teaching life? You can certainly go on as you have always done. You can even use this text as a cognitive tool and add a few more skills to your teaching tool kit. I invite you to do more with what is described here. Practice affective methods, strategies, and concepts so we can build a community of soulful teachers who want to be on this same journey.

> *Educare*, the root of the word education, means "to lead forth the hidden wholeness," the innate integrity that is in every person. And as such, there is a place where "to educate" and "to heal" means the same thing. Educators are healers. (Remen, 1999, p. 35)

It is possible you may find this journey challenging but hopefully also rewarding. We are at a place in nursing education where the average age of faculty is 56-plus years old. We have or will have significant retirements annually, and these will have a major impact on the faculty shortage over the next few years, leaving even fewer trained faculty for mentoring and teaching students and future educators. This will ultimately lead to more of a nursing shortage and there will be a desire to quickly get nurses prepared without much thought to the student nurse's affective development—a potential risk worth avoiding. *Affective Teaching in Nursing* can play an important part in future faculty development as the so-called Generation Xers come forward into the ranks of teaching nurses. This new group of educators has its own struggles in terms of being prepared to teach and bring forth affectively literate students. Imagine if our future nurse educators believed their teaching was an act of love, capable of inner maturation development, and taking on the role of a healer for our students? This type of nurse is more likely to go into the world and provide the healing needed for themselves as well as their patients.

> Since nursing is a caring profession, its ability to sustain its caring ideals, ethics, and philosophy for professional practices will affect the human development of civilization and nursing's mission in society. (Watson, 2008, p. 41)

The URLs included in this book are posted by various persons and they have the right to pull these from the Internet if and when they see fit. This may cause some links to fail in the future, and I apologize ahead of time for this inconvenience.

—Dennis Ondrejka

Acknowledgments

I worked for years on this book, but not until I worked with Vicki Bobo did I have a plan to finish. Her support and reading guidance has been the internal and external support I needed to finish this project.

I am also greatly indebted to leaders in education that have been breaking traditional educational methods and asking for a new generation of teachers. Parker Palmer, a great author and educator, has inspired me in many ways to challenge the objectivist movement as I look to integrate affective methods into the classroom. In addition, Marie Manthey and her team at Creative Health Care Management are an inspiration to us and our need to continue efforts to build relational and caring practices as nurses. It is not enough to be competent nurses, but to be passionate about how we connect to others for their best healing.

Another great educator is Jean Watson, who lives daily to change the practice of nursing to a place of presence and care. If we could just be in such a place as we meet our patients each day, we would have our inner healer moving out to all those we touch.

I also want to thank my wife, Terri, who had more sleepless nights arising from my dissertation period than from the writing of this text. However, I have had to take so much from *We Time* to be just *Me Time* and I am thankful for such a partner in my life.

PART I

The Problem in Nursing Education

Everything depends on the lenses through which we view the world. By putting on new lenses, we can see things that would otherwise remain invisible. (Palmer, 2007, p. 27)

CHAPTER 1

What Is Affective Pedagogy: What Is the Risk for Faculty?

POSSIBILITIES

As a reader of this text, walk around your college or university, visit a classroom, and look closely at the students and the teacher within. Sit for a minute in the back of the room. Challenge yourself to ignore the topic of the class, and observe only the connections that are present or absent among participants in the classroom. Don't be critical of anyone, but observe what is there. This is the reality of that particular class culture and what has been created consciously or unconsciously. You may or may not like what you see.

> It is time for us to reaffirm that education—that is teaching in all its forms—is the primary task of higher education. (Donald Kennedy, Stanford president, April 1990)

The reality is that faculty come to teaching for different reasons. Many are called to teaching as their passion, vocation, or expression of their inner selves. Others find teaching by mistake or perhaps through a confused belief that teaching is their calling. What a sad revelation it is when all a teacher can see are students who are floundering, expressing misguided thinking, or appearing inattentive and lazy. Imagine the possibilities if more faculty knew they were in the right career and their primary goal was to create a connection between themselves and their students, which worked like an umbilical cord for cognitive and affective development.

More typically, life as a nurse educator, teacher, and mentor means daily excitement as nursing students move toward independence and begin to show a connection of caring with their patients. Eventually, graduates take on the role of *becoming* a professional nurse. It is exciting to see these same students years later as they mentor new students in clinical practice. The journey is not always pleasant, friendly, or without hazards. So applaud yourself for taking the risk of becoming an educator of nurses.

What is even more worthy of recognition is a willingness to address the lost pedagogy—the affective domain. Utilizing the affective domain as pedagogy is a form of teaching that engages students in such a way that it impacts their knowledge of self, how they value or believe certain things, and it assists them in understanding the choices they make and actions they take. This approach to education transforms the student. Affective teaching has either been a mystery of meaning, or utilizing the affective domain has been too confusing for educators to incorporate into teaching practice. Nurses need a level of self-awareness to truly connect with their patients during the healing process as well as to understand their therapeutic selves. Affective teaching methods are at the core of bringing this understanding to light, and it is time to know more about what this means. This will entitle you to more than a simple acknowledgment as a teacher. It will deserve a heart-felt "thank you" for being willing to do the difficult personal work of taking a journey beyond tradition, routine, and habit to become an affective-literate teacher.

CHALLENGES OF DEFINING AFFECTIVE TEACHING

Nursing has had a wavering and poorly articulated understanding of what affective teaching or affective literacy means—even when we say that we do this as educators. Defining affective teaching is problematic, as evidenced by the wide range of descriptions available in the literature. Elizabeth King wrote *Affective Education in Nursing: A Guide to Teaching and Assessment* in 1984 as the first nursing text on the subject. She focused her work on teaching methods aimed at addressing moral value judgments for nursing, with the result being primarily an ethics development course. Her goal, however, was to have nurses develop the ability to value others as a moral way of being (King, 1984). In another description, Hammer (1990) discussed affect in terms of anything that moves into the feeling zones, which has continued to be directly correlated to the term *affect* in most literature. Beane (1990) defined affect as those aspects of humanness that involve preferences and choices. These authors described affect as having a personal, aesthetic, developmental, and cultural context. Before we have a solid understanding of how to teach toward these affective attributes, we need to value their presence within those around us, which can be called *affective literacy*. A definition that encompasses all of these authors' ideas, and for the reader's reference, affective pedagogy is:

> Through their professional priorities and in their relationships with students, professors sustain or weaken the intellectual and social environment of the college. (Boyer, 1987, p. 119)

> A form of teaching that will support the individual's integration of knowledge regarding emotion, preference, choice, feeling, belief, attitude, ethic, and personal awareness of the self.

Through this process of teaching, students will gain their own affective literacy, which will include understanding of their self-motivation for action and inaction. It will also support self-awareness regarding their behaviors and where these behaviors originate.

As a reader, this definition may seem to be more of an abstraction than a practical understanding of affective literacy. A more understandable definition of affective literacy, applied to myself is to know what motivates me; to understand why I make the choices I make; and to be in touch with my feelings and moral compass as I experience life. For example, if I am an affective-literate educator, I know when I am not connected to my students. While teaching, educators sense additional distractors present and may feel a personal emotional loss, frustration, or sadness by this disconnect. In such cases, it would be valuable for educators to look for personal or subconscious reasons for this disconnect and then accept this outcome as something they partially created.

A challenging discussion for educators is to explore the difference between why a nurse became a nurse versus why that nurse became a teacher of nursing. What are the reasons nurses become educators of nurses? Are the reasons clear and purposeful or an accident or something deeper in the affective self that has not matured enough for this understanding to be apparent? The three most common words related to low levels of self-awareness are "I don't know!" This has been a classic humorous topic for comedians like Bill Cosby (http://www.youtube.com/watch?v=8ysFvUizRj8&feature=youtu.be), but it seems less humorous when students are asked to be more reflective about what is happening to them in a clinical setting. There does appear to be an affective continuum of integration that was first acknowledged in 1964, called Bloom's Taxonomy. This taxonomy may offer some insight as to what are understandable parts of affective awareness versus what parts are still hidden.

BLOOM'S TAXONOMY AND EARLY AFFECTIVE PEDAGOGY IN NURSING

After many years of research, Krathwohl, Bloom, and Masia (1964, 1974, 1999) developed a taxonomy for objectives in education (often called Bloom's Taxonomy). The taxonomy defines the three types of learning as cognitive (mental), psychomotor (physical), and affective (emotional), with the focus of their second book on taxonomy being the affective domain. (A website that may be useful in seeing how Bloom's Taxonomy is being used today is http://www.nwlink.com/~donclark/hrd/bloom.html.) Despite significant challenges in its use, Bloom's Taxonomy has been used over the years as an aid in defining affect, understanding what might constitute a continuum of affective development, and to articulate affective development of students. Krathwohl et al.'s work helps the reader become aware of a possible maturation in terms of depth or integration of affective ideas within a certain context. They suggest five major stages in affective development. These are:

1. *Receiving*: The student becomes aware and is willing to receive the affective input.
2. *Responding*: The student begins acquiescing and exhibits a willingness to interact on this level.
3. *Valuing*: The student accepts and expresses a preference for or a commitment to the topic.
4. *Organization*: The student conceptualizes values and moves to an organized value system.
5. *Characterization by a value complex*: The student's conceptualized value complex becomes a way of life.

Overlaying a developmental continuum onto any affective concept makes the definition appear to be more fluid and offers greater challenges, but it also offers the possibility of more insight into any particular affective phenomenon. It suggests that affective learning is a developmental process, and thus, one should not expect the same level of integration to be exhibited by all students or faculty. A developmental affective continuum has significant implications for how various students and faculty perceive, integrate, and evaluate affective pedagogy and learning. However, reliable methods for assessing affective literacy based on this continuum have challenged faculty for years, preventing investigators from using the model to study affective teaching environments.

Challenges in Using Bloom's Taxonomy

In order to utilize the stages defined by Bloom's Taxonomy in affective teaching today, one must understand their weaknesses and their strengths, and be able to connect the original work to current definitions of affective learning. For example, the historic work of Krathwohl et al. (1964, 1974, 1999) mentioned earlier presents five stages of development but leaves several confusing weaknesses for investigators. Krathwohl et al.'s discussion defines *receiving* as awareness, and lacks any relationship to current affective definitions. These authors state, "Though it is the bottom rung of the affective domain, *Awareness* is almost a cognitive domain" (p. 99). It is therefore possible that *awareness* in Bloom's Taxonomy is a cognitive domain. In addition, one can make a case for the cognitive domain as part of several intermediary steps of their second level of integration called *responding*. Krathwohl et al. called the second intermediary level of responding "satisfaction in responding" (p. 118), and it makes sense to take this to the third stage on the continuum called *valuing* because this is an affective experience versus leaving it at the *responding* level, which is primarily described in cognitive terms. This means two of the five developmental levels in Bloom's Affective Taxonomy are essentially cognitive strategies. Such a theoretical discussion challenges any investigator in the use of Bloom's Affective Taxonomy for affective outcomes and measurement strategies as they were defined. In addition, the stages of *valuing, organizing,* and *the characterization of a value complex* have their own challenges that are explained by Krathwohl, Bloom, and Masia's (1999) discussion of their earlier work. These more recent discussions suggest there may be no reason to push for a separation between the affective and cognitive domains, supporting their 1964 third premise for a lack of affective objectives. They state:

> This division [cognitive, affective, and psychomotor] was found useful despite the fact that nearly all goals overlap both the cognitive and affective domains if they are stated in all of their aspects. Further, many goals extend to all three domains. The division has served to enforce the isolation of the domains from one another, to make it more difficult to unite all the aspects of a behavior into a single goal statement, and to emphasize cognitive goal aspects at the expense of others, especially the affective. (p. 197)

Krathwohl et al. believe we should let the cognitive and affective run together. They see separation as difficult now that educators are more focused on *action* outcomes that support cognitive statements regarding the course objectives. If one were to write an objective where the learner should *be able to describe . . . and value . . .,* there will still be an *action outcome* attached for the learner. In essence, the originators of the affective taxonomy are losing interest in constructing differentiating taxonomies. As Krathwohl states, "Clearly, this is a problem which will need to be considered by those who attempt the next advance of the Taxonomy" (p. 197).

The work of Freire (1998) also supports the view that cognitive and affective domains of knowing need to be integrated. He states, "We must dare so as never to dichotomize cognitive and emotion" (p. 3) as he supports a teaching style that activates a cultural change for the student. It is apparent that there is, or at least has been, a movement to eliminate the separation between affective and cognitive learning objectives that has little meaning when viewed through a certain lens.

Despite these rejections to a separation, there is value in exploring the cognitive–affective differences, as such an exploration suggests a different focus for teaching with underpinnings behind an instructor's pedagogy used in classrooms and offers a greater level of acceptance for the subjective domain. Therefore, at the outset, the separation will be a learning device, and then we can think about the blended view for future discussions. So, for the sake of building a text that promotes the affective domain of pedagogy and learning, the separation of affective and cognitive domains will continue until it serves us no longer.

FOUNDATIONS FOR AFFECTIVE PEDAGOGY

A thorough search of affective awareness strategies and learning models leads to the study of three psychological models. Psychodrama, Gestalt, and humanistic psychologies are particularly useful as a means to reach greater awareness of the intersubjective and intrasubjective selves. The constructs within these theories place great importance on affective awareness and learning related to the self, and thus provide us with ways to begin incorporating the affective domain into the classroom. Briefly, we can understand *intersubjective* as an awareness that occurs in the moment of two people connecting. It is about learning in the moment without a previous agenda. *Intrasubjective* is what we are able to learn about ourselves. It seems almost self-evident that psychological strategies might be useful in this way. Gestalt, psychodrama, and humanistic psychologies offer support for both and are foundational to affective literacy.

Psychodrama

The term *psychodrama* is believed to have been coined by Jacob Moreno (Williams, 1989). Moreno was an Austrian psychiatrist who lived from 1892 to 1976 and who is credited with the origination of group therapy. From 1909 to 1911, Moreno devised his own form of role-play, which by 1922 became a theatrical production totally structured around spontaneous work called *Das Stegreiftheater*. He initially implemented his ideas with children and later included adults who valued *being-in-the-moment-of-creation* versus pursuing goals, such as perfection. As he watched psychodrama's effect on the audiences and the actors (patients) in relation to their lives at home, Moreno wondered if the work of spontaneity could be the key to mental health (see http://www.youtube.com/watch?v=zvgnOVfLn4k&feature=youtu.be for an actual psychodrama being created by Moreno). His theatrical use of psychodrama was also highly criticized by the psychoanalytic community.

Moreno's wife, Zerka, was also very influential in the development of psychodrama strategies. Using a social systems approach, Moreno's approach was more horizontal, while Zerka favored a vertical approach that concentrated on the cathartic work that may be found by exploring primal past experiences (Fox, 1987). Zerka pulled others who had connections to the actor into the psychodrama to evaluate the dynamics being played out between them. The vertical method used by Zerka asks the actor (patient) to go inside to find the inner conflict or wound (see http://youtu.be/VQUtxDK5V-w). Williams (1989) outlines the central beliefs for using psychodrama as:

1. People have multi-role personalities.
2. Spontaneity is found in the here and now.
3. Spontaneity leads to creativity, which leads to personal awareness and healing.
4. It is action in the moment that brings about change.
5. Psychodrama fosters the creation of meaning versus the excavation of meaning found in traditional therapy.

The process of interaction between individuals, or *tele*, is critical to understanding psychodrama. The term *tele* originated from the Greek word meaning *far off*. Tele is "the simplest unit of feeling transmitted from one individual to another" (Moreno, 1953, p. 159). Kellerman (1979) described tele as the emotional feeling tone that exists in almost all human relationships. It is very similar to descriptions of intersubjective knowing or the idea of *care theory* found in more recent literature. Watson says it this way, "The meaning and essence of care are experienced in the moment when one human being connects with another" (Watson, 2004, p. viii). We continue to see our connectedness as a part of the way we experience one another, which carries on to this day.

Dayton (1994) presented psychodrama as a healing process that does not require conscious remembering of an event; the remembrance is precipitated when one's body acts out an old event. The action triggers the hidden trauma from that event but allows it to be reconstructed in the here and now with different outcomes. This is truly a subconscious learning model that allows the person who is working to re-create his or her interior life. "It provides the pathway to bring our inner and outer reality into balance and accord" (Dayton, 1994, p. 7).

It is easy to see the value of being in the moment, being open to others, creating a connection to parts of self that have another agenda, and using spontaneity and creativity to give clarity to self-awareness as useful tools for personal self-awareness and growth. The challenge is having the skills to do this in a classroom. To address this issue, let us begin to explore how psychodrama is useful in building the foundations of an affective pedagogy.

Educators often hear stories of students with math phobias, dissertation paralysis, and other traumatic academic events that play out in the student. The literature suggests that psychodrama could be used to address such issues by allowing the student (actor) to explore the old subconscious inner voice that creates his or her response. Psychodrama also provides an avenue to re-script this internal message—something that psychodramatists believe is as real as the original message in the subconscious part of the brain.

We see some of these methods in classrooms where the teacher uses a family scripting method to show family relationships (e.g., in a community health course when studying family dynamics). Imagine its use for those who fear taking tests, become paralyzed with math, or have complete loss of memory when they have to present to the class. Vignette 1.1 provides an example of just such an issue.

Vignette 1.1

I was in my first semester of college, and I needed to give a 15-minute presentation on a historical event, and I had no more than three quarters of a page of writing. I remember getting up, walking to the front of the class, but I don't remember anything else until I was sitting down. I could remember only some of what I said. I don't remember seeing a face—and at this point, I don't recall if the instructor told me anything. This became a serious inner failure in my life, and I dedicated myself to fight this type of fear forever, no matter what it took.

Two years later at a different college in California, a friend of mine and I decided to sing at a college talent night. I had been playing guitar in front of small groups and found great confidence when playing and singing. We decided to sing a Simon and Garfunkel song, "Scarborough Fair." We knew the audience would be around 5,000 people who would also vote on us in relation to other presentations. It was then that I realized I found power and self-esteem when holding a guitar and singing. It was freeing to know I could find a way to be confident in front of thousands of people—and share a part of myself.

Would it be possible to gain such awareness about oneself in a classroom? Maybe it would work for presentation anxiety, or test anxiety if we had alternative ways to present things creatively. What if we used poems, music, or other ways to address these challenging issues for students?

Gestalt Psychology

Another theory that places great importance on affective awareness and learning related to the self is Gestalt psychology. Heidbreder (1933) wrote about the development of Gestalt perspectives at the turn of the 20th century and at its origination by Max Wertheimer in 1910. Wertheimer became convinced there was something wrong with the explanations of sensory processes and perception available to him at the time, so he looked for an alternative. His original concern was the fundamental problem of clinicians and scientists not addressing how a phenomenon is perceived, described, and interpreted. Two students of Wertheimer, Wolfgang Kohler and Kurt Koffka, also became convinced of the inadequacy of the *older psychology* that bore the *Wundtian* stamp of approval. In response, these three men initiated a protest movement called Gestalt psychology, which had no equivalent translation in the English language. Gestalt more recently has been defined as "to make a comprehensive whole" (Hardy, 1991, p. 4) and has been influenced by the work of Fritz Perls. "Gestalt therapy is a philosophy that tries to be in harmony, in alignment with everything else—with medicine, with science, with the universe, with what is" (Perls, 1969, pp. 16–17). Perls also taught classes on what it meant to be using Gestalt (see http://www.youtube.com/watch?v=T3jYcDbcpUs&feature=youtu.be).

Hardy's (1991) discussion of Gestalt therapy covers several central beliefs concerning the universality of the theory:

1. Man is a mind–body connection that cannot be separated.
2. Gestalt therapy emphasizes the person's self-regulation by enhanced awareness.

3. It aims to bring into awareness these polarities of the human experience in order to enhance completeness and spontaneity.
4. It strongly supports experiential learning.
5. It supports equilibrium between society and personal goals by all persons who are living in concerned contact with their environments.
6. It places great importance on learning that problem solving is a process rather than an end itself.
7. Experiencing a feeling is the most effective way to meet Gestalt therapy objectives.
8. It addresses feelings and concepts in the here-and-now and rejects the value of describing things or giving a historical view.

As we explore affective teaching methods, it is clear how such issues become foundational philosophies for the faculty member who strives for affective literacy in his or her students. In some cases it brings out exceptional creativity that also can become aligned with learning (see *The Cosby Show* video clip: http://www.youtube.com/watch?v=5-2NmLTdSq8).

Carl Jung also influenced Gestalt therapy, but Gestalt psychologists revised Jung's polarity concepts to develop the idea of *being-in-paradox*. Gestalt therapists asserted that any part of the self has a counterpart, and this counterpart is what Gestalt therapists use for self-awareness and development by asking the client to respond to a potential concern that is 180 degrees from what they started with—the paradox question. Thus, if the client is concerned about struggling with a relationship, the counterpart work of the client would be to ask what would it be like right now if everything was perfect for him or her in the relationship. If this can be articulated, then an outcome goal has just been created. If it cannot be articulated, then the struggle is (a) to get clarity and (b) to realize that both the positive and the negative issues can be real for the client.

This philosophy supports personal responsibility for one's feelings, behaviors, and choices even if they are creating a paradox for the self, which are also major outcomes of affective literacy. In Gestalt therapy, the use of transference, or redirecting emotions to the therapist in order to work through an issue, is avoided because it creates dependency on the therapist rather than promoting the notion of taking responsibility for one's own improvement.

Gestalt practitioners (Beisser, 1970; Hardy, 1991; Perls, 1972) repeatedly predict that clients (and possibly students) will become healthier as they become who they really are rather than continuing their attempts to be someone else. Sometimes this is described as wearing a mask at work, a different mask when a student, and another mask when home with family. The challenge is to have such an in-depth level of awareness that we can really see who we are and not need all the masks. Faculty members who are learning about their inner selves and how their assumptions impact their teaching, have been challenged to find his or her authentic self. Certain types of reflection methods are aimed directly at this sense of self. We often ask students to be reflective of who they were trying to be in a given situation, and how that is working for them. Both are examples of Gestalt processes.

Humanistic (Rogerian) Therapy

Humanistic therapy also has great value in building a foundation for affective awareness and learning. The work of Carl Rogers as a humanistic psychologist is well known in the field of psychology and education. His earlier work was specific to the therapeutic relationship (Rogers, 1951), which fostered self-initiated action, flexibility, use of personal experiences, and client-centered openness. Rogers's work (1969) was also directed at an inner connection between facilitator and learner, and states, "Certain attitudinal qualities which exist in the personal relationship between the facilitator and the learner, produce significant learning" (p. 106). The goal is to view the world through your student's eyes. Rogers's *person-centered* methods in education require teachers to be flexible, transparent, collaborative with the students, and to support student self-evaluation. (A clip of Carl Rogers providing humanistic therapy support, which is highly patient-centered, can be found at http://www.youtube.com/watch?v=m30jsZx_Ngs.)

The recent research of Cornelius-White (2007) has identified humanistic educational practices as primary strategies for creating *learner-centered* teachers who build positive relationships with their students. His meta-analysis suggests that teachers who are empathetic to student needs positively impact student outcomes. This occurs when teachers provide unconditional positive regard, are genuine, are less directing, and ask for more critical thinking.

The historical development and practice of Gestalt psychology, psychodrama, and humanistic therapy laid a foundation for connecting affective literacy to self-awareness. These psychological therapies have basic constructs that are equally effective beliefs and techniques for fostering the in-depth personal awareness that may be made apparent in various affective learning environments. However, it has been historically unclear how well affective learning works for students or what are the pedagogical factors necessary to make it a successful learning experience.

Ways of Knowing

In addition to building a foundation for affective pedagogy, it is important to understand how we learn, otherwise known as ways of knowing. Carper's (1978) ground-breaking work that was expanded by Jacobs-Kramer and Chinn (1992) describes four classical critical thinking domains frequently used to categorize types of learned experiences: *aesthetic*, *ethical*, *personal*, and *empirical* domains of knowing. In addition, the literature suggests a fifth way of knowing that is called *intersubjective* knowing (Crossley, 1996; Munhall, 1993; Watson, 2008). This foundational look at how we learn, creates a framework for understanding all types of academic strategies. The affective domain is especially correlated to the aesthetic, ethical, personal, and intersubjective domains. Understanding the ways of knowing may not be a foundation for creating affective pedagogy, but it certainly helps explain how various types of teaching differ as well as how the student is impacted and matures.

The aesthetic domain includes artistic and intuitive types of knowing. It encompasses the personal interpretation of art, music, drama, and natural phenomena, such as being in the woods. The individual experiences his or her own personal interpretation of that process, and that interpretation can be used to examine how he or she connects to others within an aesthetic experience.

The ethical domain includes values, morals, and personal belief structures that are core decision-making frameworks within the individual. Much of this learning occurs early in life and is then carried into adulthood as a value structure. In some cases, academic settings attempt to shape this part of the person's knowing by addressing service, professional empathetic relationships, or constructs related to professional ethics.

The personal domain is the knowledge gained from personal experiences in life or in a personal problem-solving strategy called *heuristic* knowing. It encompasses skills or even specialized personal awareness strategies commonly identified as *experience-based learning* that occurs outside any formal academic setting. It is possible to see this type of knowing as growth-enhancing or growth-stunting, where the latter believes the only valued knowledge is from personal experience and the rest is not real.

Empirical knowing includes the scientific method and research knowledge. It is described as a rational or cognitive way of knowing. The academic setting is typically credited with providing empirical knowing, which is often seen as the best or most likely truth. The idea that empirical inquiry offers the most accurate or best truth about a topic is based on our culture's deeply held belief regarding the usefulness of validity and reliability in structuring scientific inquiry. Despite its empirical credibility, it is only one of five domains of knowing described in this text, which can also be used to assess pedagogy and learning.

The fifth domain of knowing is called intersubjective knowing, which encompasses the work of Mead, Cooley, and Blumer and their descriptions of symbolic interaction, symbolic introspection, and sympathetic introspection, respectively (Mayers, 2003; Polkinghorne, 1983; Prus, 1996). Intersubjective knowing represents a type of knowing that only occurs as two or more people come together and create a new level of awareness not understood by the participants individually before they interacted. Watson (2008) put it this way, "Learning is more than receiving information, facts, or data. It involves a meaningful, trusting relationship that is intersubjective; the nature of the relationship as well as the form and content of teaching affects the process" (p. 125). Munhall's (1993) description of a nurse showing up in the *unknowing* is a useful way of thinking about how we learn when not having an agenda already present. She challenges us to withhold our beliefs, personal ideas, projections, and biases to have a better understanding of what is happening in the moment. It is important to note that a nursing researcher such as Munhall was looking at a very subjective topic in the early 1990s as a way to learn more. The idea is identical to the former authors who wrote about the "intersubjective knowing methods." Again, it is about being present, without your own understanding of the issues before you, until you are in connection with the other person. This creates the new "intersubjective" knowing.

These five ways of knowing help us build a framework for understanding academic strategies. By understanding how students learn, we can begin to build a foundation for affective approaches to teaching. To arrive at a clear and complete framework, though, we need to understand our ways of knowing in conjunction with social–emotional learning (SEL) and how this plays out with intersubjective experiences.

Social–Emotional Learning

Most of the SEL educational models and research are used in K–12 settings where there is a need to instill competencies and skill development in young children and young adults as a way to improve socialization abilities. There is some research on using these skills in adult classrooms as well as a way for teachers and students to learn to work together more effectively. Such work is closely tied to affective literacy for teachers and social–emotional literacy for teachers and students. However, there is a significant cognitive component in how SEL is being used in many other settings that again represents the difficulty theorists have in separating the affective from the cognitive as we explore the topic of affective literacy.

> The emphasis on emotional skills reveals that emotion per se is not the focus; rather, it is the cognitive processing of emotion that is important—the "reasoning about" emotion and the behaviors one associated with such reasoning. SEL is fundamentally about psychometric and pedagogical possibility: Skills can be taught and the learner's competence in their performance can be measured. (Hoffman, 2009, p. 538)

Hoffman (2009) identified several purely cognitive models in practice that were aimed at producing measurable outcomes for students learning SEL. He states that this emphasis on skill and cognitive processing of emotions has been seen as a valuable outcome of successful SEL training of students who are going into the world or beginning their careers (Cohen, 2006; Goleman, 1995; Stern, 2007). It also points to the challenges of staying true to the need to measure the subjective. Of greater concern in this review of SEL is how teachers might use, model, and mentor such skills as living proof of their value in the classroom, if they do use such strategies.

Faculty who are teaching adults have additional challenges. Adult students have already formed many opinions regarding education, their need to learn (or not), whether you are a good teacher (or not), and may have a host of reasons for being in that course—ranging from the excitement of learning to a boredom that is tied to a required course for their major. No longer are you dealing with SEL methods as a proper way to ask for help on an assignment. SEL can easily become a technique to teach rather than a community norm of activity based on Hoffman's research. Palmer (2007) puts it this way: "Good teaching cannot be reduced to technique; good teaching comes from the identity and integrity of the teacher" (p. 10). He relates this to knowing yourself as a teacher and that you are "willing to make it available and vulnerable in the service of learning" (p. 10).

SEL addresses the affective in many ways and higher education can take lessons from what we have seen for 20 years in K–12 settings. However, we must still heed the experts from these programs:

> I am a bit bothered by the great emphasis in current research on teaching the kids social skills such as listening. Of course it is important for students to learn how to listen and treat one another with some sensitivity, but it is also important that teachers listen to the students. (Nodding, 2006, p. 239)

This is the real essence of using SEL in higher education. It allows for the intersubjective experience where the student and teacher learn together in the cognitive and affective domains.

The foundations of affective pedagogy incorporate elements from all the areas discussed earlier. An understanding of the three psychological theories outlined here (psychodrama, Gestalt, and humanistic therapy) provides us with affective awareness strategies and learning models. Further, an understanding of our ways of knowing and SEL bring forward how intersubjective experiences impact the cognitive and affective domains. Now we will use this foundational knowledge to begin exploring ways in which we can use affective pedagogy in the classroom.

CONTEMPORARY EDUCATION THEORIES AND AFFECTIVE PEDAGOGY

> Teachers in classrooms often rely heavily on automated presentation software and use pedagogical strategies that are significantly less effective than teachers generally use in clinical settings and skills labs, where knowledge acquisition use is more integrated. (Benner, Sutphen, Leonard, & Day, 2010, p. 65)

Affective pedagogy may be designed specifically by the instructor to address particular types of knowing. In addition, classroom cultures can be examined through theories of effective teaching called *care pedagogy*, *teacher immediacy*, and *pedagogical typology*, and the physical classroom structure called *proxemics*. Other approaches to affective pedagogy have come from student learning styles and have focused on how the student can create his or her own learning method.

Contemporary Educational Theories

This section provides curriculum development theories that allow the reader to understand where various forms of curricula originate. Some curriculum models make affective pedagogy easier to apply, and there are examples of how they come together. In other cases, a certain curriculum philosophy would not be used to build affective teaching methods. Having educational theories as a landscape allows the reader to determine how to use them in more critical and intentional ways, especially when looking to bring in affective methods.

Bertrand's (2003) work on contemporary education theories provides a comprehensive discussion of what American educators have used as the foundation for building curricula. There are obviously other ways to categorize our educational history, and we will explore some of these as well. However, using Bertrand's categorization, the first trend for American educators originated from the desire to teach and create teaching theories around solid pillars of knowledge called *academic theories.*

Academic Theories

The role of the teacher involves the dissemination of content around well-known topics such as liberal arts, classical literature, the sciences, and mathematics. These were called the *academic theories*, and they were given descriptive names such as classical, generalist, functionalist, traditionalist, and pragmatist. In the academic theories, each student is tasked with complying with competency-based education. There is no room for questioning the norms of social standards in these theories. The process is highly prescriptive and cognitive without any flexibility in approach because the teacher has the expertise and the content is archetypal and transcends time, leaving students to be more passive and simply hear and *get it.*

There are some variances within the global domain of academic theories. These variations, or subcategories, still are in alignment with the premise of what an academic theory is—to pass on to the next generation key and everlasting principles. The first subcategory is *classical theories*, which asks the student to hear classical content that is void of current culture or changes within the current social fabric. In nursing, an example might be the belief that nurses should show patients a conservative outer look—no visible tattoos, minimal ear piercing, and no facial piercing. In an age where these classical principles may not hold up, we may face the potential need to re-think such principles. However, it wasn't long ago that these classical messages in nursing were that a nurse should wear a white uniform, white shoes, a nurse's cap, and a nurse's pin. Where did these classical messages go? It is an interesting question to ask.

A second subcategory of academic theories as posited by Bertrand (2003) is called the *generalist theories.* In this domain, the instructors stress a certain way of thinking through problems and focus on our logical minds creating rational solutions to complex issues. It also involves the critical and open mind that does not have a purely biased preconception of what is occurring. Let us look at the nursing process as our method of integrating the genera-list theories approach. Nurses collect the data that can be objective and subjective, and then assess this to meet a logical conclusion regarding the patient's problem from a nursing perspective. The nurses give it a diagnosis that is open to nursing interventions and then intervene using these learned methods from the profession. The diagnosis is evaluated to see if the intervention(s) worked and make adjustments to have the best patient outcomes. Vinette 1.2 shows what nursing looks like within a generalist theory process.

Vignette 1.2

Data Collection:

Mr. Marks, 64 years old, was admitted 2 days ago. He was previously diagnosed with congestive heart failure, hypertension, and cardiac ischemic injury in 1990. He is currently complaining of intermittent chest pain occurring for the past week. He has allergies to sulfa drugs. In the emergency department he had an EKG, which was negative, and his troponin levels were twice normal. He recently worked on his house, building a deck. He had erythemic bed pressure spots on the buttock and scapula when he arrived to the unit. He has been in the emergency department for 12 hours.

He has a peripheral line in the right forearm that is patent with normal saline running at 40 mL/hr, with a Lasix piggyback drip running that was started 30 minutes earlier. Urine is normal now, but is very concentrated.

Vital signs on admission to the unit were BP 140/88, P 52, T 98.8, R 28, pulse-ox 90%; he is still complaining of chest pain intermittently. Potassium levels are 3.0 and he has 2+ pitting edema in the lower legs and feet. Reduced breath sounds in lower lung lobes, normal breath sounds in upper lung fields. Heart has a normal rhythm.

Medication order includes:

Nitro tabs sublingual, as needed for chest pain every 2 hours

Beta blocker every day

Motrin 600 every 6 hours as needed for pain

Lasix 20 mEq in 100-cc bag, piggybacks, IV three times a day

Oxygen is by cannula at 6 liters

Nursing Diagnoses:

1. Intermittent chest pain related to ineffective fluid mobilization in lungs and interstitial spaces related to cardiac insufficiency
2. Poor skin integrity related to poor circulation and stagnant positioning

Nurse Interventions:

1. Provide skin care, and move patient to right side using pillows
2. Check for good oxygenation and cannula placement
3. Hold beta blocker until pulse is up to 60 bpm and call physician

(continued)

4. Call physician for potassium order and indwelling Foley as the Lasix kicks in; discuss the possible use of a daily 85 mg aspirin and when to get another troponin and potassium blood level
5. Assess leg edema every 8 hours, get an accurate patient weight, and monitor every 8 hours
6. Turn the patient side to side every 2 hours or get special padding mattress, then check and treat skin every 2 hours

Nurse Evaluations:

1. Vital signs every 4 hours with weight every 8 hours
2. Intake and output monitoring
3. Skin monitoring every 2 hours
4. Ask the patient his perception of ease of breathing, pain, and skin needs
5. Recheck troponin and potassium levels
6. Discuss any changes with the physician, especially fluid retention, potassium dropping, or poor urine output

As illustrated in Vignette 1.2, a generalist theory is a useful approach in nursing to integrate the nursing process, which includes data collection, assessment, nursing interventions, evaluation, and any necessary adjustments. Most nurses have experienced the generalist theory approach and, over time, have certainly become better at this straightforward technique. However, the approach is void of relational knowledge—the subjective elements involving the patient's self-motivation or self-care deficits.

Bertrand (2003) also presents another subcategory of academic theories called *functionalist theories*, where there is more of an attempt at having the student show competency in his or her actions as a professional in any setting or situation in American society. Nursing has used this concept to provide the nurse with professional strategies of success, a skill set normally saved for the baccalaureate educational level of nursing. It has been called *leadership* or *professional practice*, and often provides the nurse with the principles for professional practice such as being patient centered and a patient advocate. These principles will always allow the nurse to function in a way that is acceptable in American society and are represented in Figure 1.1, which shows patient-centered care.

It is a complex issue to examine the usefulness of each subgroup of academic theories in conjunction with affective pedagogy. However, it is possible that all three of the academic theories described here could use affective methods to get the information to the student, although this would not be likely, as the theories are primarily teacher- or curriculum-focused. The academic theories may serve as a mirror of your practice or may provide some understanding of teaching methods not being used when presenting affective pedagogy. As a student of educational methods, there is value in learning both.

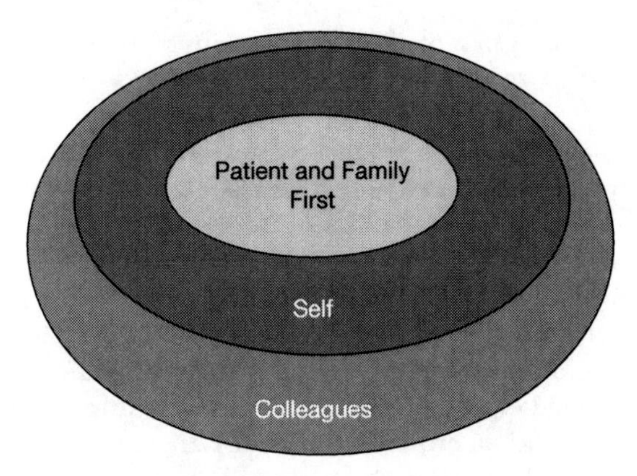

The CORE of the healing environment is your relationship to the patient and family

Figure 1.1 Nurse advocacy model.
Modified from Koloroutis (2004).

Learning Environment Theories

The *learning environment theories* focus on different constructs within the educational system that include the student, society, and the content being taught. These theories flow from the psychological theories of learning, which include cognitive theories, social cognitive theories, and instructional system design theories (Bertrand, 2003). The first of these is purely cognitive, but can be thought of as "internal processes of the mind. . . [or] a development of learning abilities and strategies" (p. 13). Cognitive theories are difficult to examine separately from other issues going on for the student, especially in nursing education. The overall nursing curriculum is intended to build internal processes for thinking through increasingly complex clinical situations, as the student moves from course to course. Cognitive theories seem too encompassing to be thought of as a teaching theory; rather, they seem to be a way of thinking about curriculum.

The second subcategory of learning environment theories is called *social cognitive theory*. This asks students to be conscious of the social and cultural interactions that occur during their educational experience. Social cognitive theory focuses on teaching and learning through various forms of social interaction, which has the potential for being highly affective even in the most traditional teaching environments—it must be experiential and affective or learning would not occur. Social cognitive approaches imply social interaction–connection–awareness of social and cultural similarities and differences. Nursing students who travel to other countries or have certain community health experiences can have their affective development impacted significantly.

The third subcategory of the learning environment theories is called *instructional systems design theories*; these again are focused on the larger picture of the curriculum. An example would be a system that states when to start the clinical experience and when to have prerequisite course requirements, and it would ask questions such as, "Is it effective to have specialty nursing training, for example, pediatrics, prior to completing all the medical-surgical courses?" The large domain of instructional systems design theories encompasses when and how to use technology, simulation, clinical placement, lab practice, video, DVD, television, and webinar. It becomes developmental when it is used to capture the learning styles of various students and helps determine how they would be most successful. For affective literacy, it is a critical domain for all persons involved in creating curricula so as to include how teaching would be taught using various forms of affective pedagogy. One simple strategy for integrating affective teaching into media is to show a film (e.g., *The Doctor* http://www.imdb.com/title/tt0101746/?ref_=sr_3) and then have nurses or student nurses provide critical reflection regarding how they interpreted the message from various perspectives.

Social Theories

The third domain of Bertrand's (2003) educational theories is the *social theories*. These theories hold to a belief that education can and "ought to allow us to resolve social, cultural, and environment problems" (p. 15). These theories have laid the groundwork for social justice in nursing, ecological awareness, and social intelligence content in many academic programs. The first subcategory for social theories is *critical pedagogy theories*, which looks at the use of power and power differentials in various cultures or in a social structure. This domain is often addressed within nursing related to nurse–physician dynamics by including games and role play. Current nursing academic environments give very little didactic time to the subject even if it is a major issue for nurses in practice today. It takes some very special personal learning and awareness for a faculty member to address the social theories because they are a relatively new level of consciousness for American society, especially in nursing. It is still uncommon for most faculty members to understand the depth of critical pedagogy theory as provided by Freire (1970, 2009), because historically it has been the nurse–physician dynamic that has been discussed. But the theory could be applied in any delegation role (e.g., a nurse working with a certified nursing assistant or a licensed practical nurse). It can be seen between management and staff and in the entire language used in the growing institutional nursing practice model called *shared governance*. In terms of teaching assessment, we will examine critical reflection as a key method that assesses how much power we use in the classroom. Vignette 1.3 is an example of how we might use critical reflection in connection with a Gestalt technique.

Vignette 1.3

Well, how did I deal with "power" in class today? I showed authoritative power in discussion of an experimental research design. I was specific, maybe dictatorial, in my knowing of the three elements needed in such a design. I then gave examples of such designs. I also dispersed power as the student groups went out to critique their section of the experimental study. When they came back to discuss their group critique of their specific section, I added my perceptions as a member of each group. Our combined critique of the content areas seemed to bring up several discussions regarding such designs. I hoped to share the power of our findings as we all contributed to the collective critique.

So my assumptions were that no one would read the content on experimental designs until we discussed it in class first. I assumed the content seemed too abstract unless grounded in examples, and only then would reading the content from the text add value to what was heard in this course—which I believe is unique to teaching research. I assumed I could contribute and reduce my power base as the instructor. Actually, I don't believe this method made my life easier as an instructor, because I had to be constantly aware of how I interacted with each group as we created the collective critique in class. I believe I was not too authoritative with each group and provided balanced input for each group to prevent the perception that some students had more of my input than others.

I do wonder about expressing my opinions when they differ from the text. I want to keep tabs on that inner discussion.

One Step Back *(a Gestalt technique, emphasizing self-regulation for deeper awareness)*

So if I step back one step from my reflective note above, I should be even more aware of what was going on for me in that class today. I would say that I wrote my critical reflection note about a teaching experience into which I put significant effort. I felt good about it when it was over. I avoided reflecting on the parts of the class that were not received as favorably. WOW! I like to talk about my positive experiences, but maybe I'm avoiding my growth area? Next time, I will reflect on a class that seemed to go badly for me.

Two Steps Back *(going deeper)*

Okay, for all of you who are ready to integrate the "hidden" or "shadow" side of self, I have a powerful reflection tool for you. Take one more step back from your reflection note and reflect on what you said in the "one-step-back" section. The first step is "Why I wrote what I wrote versus what I did not write" to give me more self-awareness. This next step can move me to my unconscious self. It is asking, "What is it about me that made me choose what I chose," and then look at the meaning at a core level. So here goes. . . .

I think I chose a positive example because I want to feel good about myself and my teaching. I can't stand the thought of writing a textbook on effective teaching and then show my readers I can be a power-hungry person in the classroom—which I could actually do, I have done it. Am I really ready to become this self-aware?

In Vignette 1.3 one can see the use of critical pedagogy theory in practice and how the foundations of affective teaching apply to bring enhanced and deeper awareness to the teacher.

The second subcategory of social theories called *learning community theories* asks the student to have personal growth in combination with his or her social awareness and involvement. There are many constructs in this domain that are perfectly aligned with affective teaching and learning. It involves the use of teams, groups, and cooperative instruction that looks for outcomes in social skills. This theory is a perfect fit for SEL models, discussed earlier.

The third subcategory is *ecosocial theories,* where there is a focus on a need to address the interaction between humans and their environment. The concern is an ecological one, one that is global, serious, and being integrated more frequently into nursing curricula. It most often comes to a school of nursing by a younger, socially aware population of students that have already placed this factor into their lives in a permanent way. Now, as nurses, they bring this forward as a way of being, rather than an educational process. Faculty continue to expand this form of care for more than just the people we care for, rather for the world we live in. Again, it is worth stating that each of the social theories requires self-aware nurses who bring most of this information along with them from their prenursing past to change the environments in which they are learning. It may also involve an enlightened faculty member who has intentionally made these new and necessary changes in his or her teaching, so that even his or her language is different. Such teachers often live this way as a natural way of being in the world and bring it into the classroom as if it were a given and known to everyone in the room. In other cases, it is not in the consciousness of the faculty member and is rarely discussed. Certainly in the past 10 years we see more of the social theories come to life in nursing, and we will probably have seen more as the next generation of faculty brings to the classroom topics of power differentials, personal awareness, social change, and ecology.

Humanistic Theories

The final group of theories presented by Bertrand (2003) are the *humanistic theories*, which include *self-awareness theories*, *dynamic interaction theories*, and *spiritual theories.* Each of these domains is easily taught using affective pedagogy and each also runs directly into the challenges addressed earlier regarding the interface between education and psychotherapy. In fact, these theories come from the world of humanistic psychology, dynamic psychology, psychoanalysis, group interaction, and spiritual self-understanding. The first subcategory is called self-actualization theories and is fully integrated into the affective and subjective domains of the student. It is focused on the internal dynamics of needs, desires, impulses, and energy of the person. It would be impossible to tell a student to feel a certain way, but faculty would be able to facilitate this process if trained to do so. One method might be to ask students certain self-awareness questions at the start of the first class and then ask the same questions at the end of the course to look at what might be occurring for them related to knowing the self.

The second subcategory for this group of theories is called dynamic interaction theories, which is ". . .mainly affective consequences of these interactions on the individual. . . . The principle is quite simple: learning is deeply 'affected' by feelings, emotions, actions, and values generated by interactions within a small group, classroom, family, . . . etc." (Bertrand, 2003, pp. 16–17). The essence of this approach is affective pedagogy and learning. The self-awareness developed in this form of teaching is important and obvious, as presented in this text.

The last subcategory for Bertrand's humanistic theories is called spiritual theories, a very interesting concept for nursing education. In faith-based institutions, the spiritual domain is addressed in various ways either as an outcome of how one lives his or her life in service to God or how one lives the spiritual values of social caring and justice. Some institutions may be based on metaphysics or may make their spiritual beliefs more integral to the curriculum, with courses in energy work or quantum physics. They may have an eclectic concept of a power greater than ourselves as a way to stay focused on the spiritual needs of others and society. Watson (1989) embodies this metaphysical awareness, and she states, "Because of the human nature of nursing, its moral, spiritual, and metaphysical components cannot be ignored. These components are inherent in the nursing process . . ." (p. 220). Watson (2008) continues this belief today in her work on integrating the 10 Caritas Processes, with number 10 stating that we should be "opening and attending to spiritual mysterious, unknown existential dimensions, of life–death–suffering; allowing for a miracle" (p. 31). Figure 1.2 is a representation of Bertrand's theories integrated into one model.

To summarize the contemporary theory model, one can identify how large, diverse curriculum templates impact the actual teaching strategy within them. It is possible to identify how one can integrate a method of teaching such as affective methods into almost all the subcategories presented. This is something one might examine when ready to construct such teaching methods in one's current practice.

HOLISTIC CURRICULUM MODELS

Some education curriculum models have been defined as *holistic*. Such theorists believe in the ability to integrate comprehensive learning using broad-reaching course objectives that originate from thinking about the whole student and all his or her learning needs. In one holistic curriculum model, Mayes (2003) examines curricula from seven different *landscapes* that connect philosophy, developmental student needs, and strategies. He calls them:

1. Organisimic landscape
2. Transferential landscape

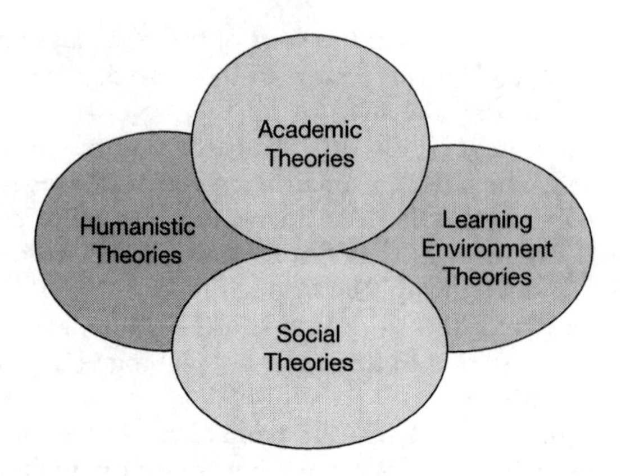

Figure 1.2 Bertrand theories of practice in education, 2003.
Adapted by Ondrejka.

3. Concrete affiliative landscape
4. Interpretive–procedural landscape
5. Phenomenological landscape
6. Unitive–spiritual landscape
7. Dialectic–spiritual landscape

Not all of these holistic teaching approaches will serve the reader of this text; these various landscapes are heavily woven into philosophy and would take significant time to understand and then use in the world of affective teaching within nursing. However, Mayes's *phenomenological landscape* offers significant points in relation to affective teaching. Mayes's (2003) discussion is highly complex, but it is possible to see the potential for how affective strategies are foundational in the curriculum and instruction that is imbedded into the aesthetic–phenomenological characteristics. He discusses Maslow, Dewey, Greene, and Nodding, addressing some aspect of *self-realization* within the educational system using the aesthetic–phenomenological approach. Nursing has used aesthetics such as poetry, film, music, case studies, and pictures for many years as a means for creating self-awareness on the part of students. It has also been used for more complex awareness as found in intersubjective knowing. All of these approaches are explored in depth later in the text.

RISK FOR AFFECTIVE TEACHERS

The following sections discuss the risks that an affective teacher takes in some academic settings. These risks are primarily professional in nature, and many are the result of political issues within higher education as well as the perceptions of faculty members of academic freedom. Given the nature of affective teaching and its ties to self-reflection and self-understanding, there is also value in examining whether a teacher is providing affective education or therapy in a classroom. Thus, it should be noted that although there are risks in teaching affectively, there are also potential ways to mitigate these risks via the approach in the classroom.

Various risks have been discussed for faculty who pursue affective forms of teaching, and some research exists for how it has been addressed in different classroom settings. In an earlier writing (Ondrejka, 1998), it was found that faculty and students both recognized that faculty are taking some degree of professional risk when engaging in affective teaching.

There also appears to be a political component that influences affective teaching methods. The *Chronicle of Higher Education* has published several historical cases, one at Colby College where the department gave the instructor in question tenure with a 4 to 1 vote. Later, the tenure committee overruled the decision with a 3 to 6 vote because of angry letters sent to the administration from some students. Defenders of the educator were very outspoken when they said, "Colby got rid of him because administrators were worried about angering parents, who pay close to $30,000 annually for their children to attend the college" (Leatherman, Nov. 1, 1996, p. A13). In this case, the professor lost, and it was directly related to his affective teaching style.

At Oakland Community College, another educator received an administrative complaint and a charge of sexual harassment from a student who felt his teaching methods were offensive and "X-rated" (Wilson, December 12, 1997, p. A14). His direct discussion of various psychological phenomena, such as the castration anxiety theory of Freud, were topics that created the controversy. Because of previous complaints by students, this educator provided the class with a written disclaimer, stating, "If controversial concepts and words bother you, be forewarned" (p. A14). This disclaimer was his attempt to warn students about the presentation of certain human phenomena that are currently labeled "politically incorrect." In the past, students opted for another section of this course if they disliked this teaching style. Given the current social climate, however, it is not too surprising that the recent student complaint was related to discussions of sexuality or some aspect of sexual thought with no self-accountability for his or her inner underpinnings for such discomfort.

Spitzberg (1987) presented a host of political pressures that can influence the curriculum as a control or expansion mechanism. His discussion is not optimistic regarding curricular innovations because of a steady undercurrent of conservatism within educational institutions in general. Spitzberg reported Kerr's view that more rapid change will occur through the development of new institutions with different views and missions, arguing that we should not expect current institutions to make anything other than iterative changes. These conservative views certainly provide a perspective of risk for faculty who might threaten the stability of funding, influential families, or even the mainstream of income from the students themselves by implementing innovative changes that address affective literacy.

Affective Education or Therapy?

There seem to be conflicting arguments about making a classroom appear as a therapy session or the view that a classroom is a place of therapeutic development and growth. A major risk to faculty who use affective pedagogy is directly related to this conflict. Students are able to exert significant pressure to stop a class from dealing with their inner growth and inner awareness issues. Some students demand that faculty be purely objective, and stay away from any affective educational methods. In 1977, William Kirman wrote *Modern Psychoanalysis in the Schools* because he believed it was needed to address all the unconscious issues and motivators found in the academic system. He believed students needed to look at these psychological issues at the elementary, secondary, and university levels. Most affective educators would agree.

Could it be that the risk of providing affective education is the very reason we believe it is needed—and resisted? The originator of rational–emotive therapy (RET) certainly saw a connection when he said, "rational–emotive therapy procedures are closely connected to the field of education and have enormous implications for emotional prophylaxis" (Ellis, 1989, p. 223). Is it possible that affective education has the same outcome desires as psychotherapy? An exploration of the two types of outcomes as shown in Table 1.1 should give reason for pause and may suggest that educators finally decide—should we provide classroom therapy in our teaching?

One may hear that students today are narcissistic, have external loci of control, are emotionally thwarted, resist any form of self-awareness, have low levels of maturity, are obsessive–compulsive, and are self-absorbed and inflexible. What happened to the thinking that suggests students are self-motivated, adult learners, seekers of knowledge, growth-oriented, flexible, and resilient partners in a learning-centered environment? Most educators have felt both sides, and there are times when they struggle with staying positive in their thinking about students.

Imagine being open and direct about what you would like education to do for all those who attend learning-centered educational programs. What if psychotherapy outcomes were a natural and mutually accepted process in every classroom? Do some students resist with lawsuits and condemnation of a faculty member who uses affective education in his or her learning environment because affective education seems to have the same outcomes as psychotherapy? It is easy to see why there can be resistance, and in many cases, it is resisted with a vengeance. This raises two critical issues for those providing affective teaching. First, not everyone will find the processes acceptable, and there are potential risks associated with the educational model. Second, it may be wise to use less invasive or introspective ways of

Table 1.1 Comparison of Affective Outcomes and Psychotherapy Outcomes

Affective Education Outcomes	Psychotherapy Outcomes
Self-awareness	Build self-esteem, acceptance, and self-awareness
Personal growth	Better growth and achievement of potential
Create a learner–teacher partnership	Provide empathy and unconditional positive regard
Get in touch with one's emotions	Be in touch with one's feelings and still be able to function effectively
Build in a self-reflective learning process	Promote actualized tendencies to support persons to be all they can be
Know your personal barriers and blocks	Rebuild one's self-valuing system with healthier ones that reshape the self
Better awareness of others as different or the same	Build a persona of positive self-regard
Develop better balance and flexibility	Shifting the client from rigid modes to those that are more open and flexible
Have increased coping and conflict resolution ability	To best see one's behavior, one needs to learn from internal awareness
Have a better life	

Source: Adapted from Corsini and Wedding (2011).

conducting affective learning that will not easily be compared to the idea of having psychotherapy in the classroom. Teachers may consider methods that slowly build on self-awareness and provide alternatives to those who resist such learning.

The illusion of academic tolerance is a thread that has woven its way through our educational institutions from its conception (Duryea, 1987). The illusion is one of complete academic freedom that is sometimes identified as being synonymous with faculty autonomy. Duryea suggests that the two concepts are very different. Significant historical analysis (Kaplan & Schrecker, 1983; McConnell, 1987; Olswang & Lee, 1984; Slaughter, 1987) and legal cases of the 1990s (Leatherman, 1996; O'Neil, 1996; Wilson, 1997) suggest that faculty do not have complete freedom or autonomy to teach what and how they wish. However, the risks vary and are related to the institution and the social climate at the time. Perhaps the climate for classroom innovation is finally improving.

SUMMARY

The literature supports the idea of fostering affective literacy in higher education settings. Although this goal is not universally accepted, many authors see this process as an ethical responsibility and believe faculty should be accountable for the holistic development of their students. This chapter provides the reader with a brief introduction to the origins of ways to examine teaching pedagogy with an emphasis on how they connect to affective methods. These methods challenge the reader to envision how these high-impact strategies might be used in the classroom.

Integrating multiple theoretical teaching frameworks provides the reader with a comprehensive platform from which to explore affective pedagogy beyond the simplistic view of method alone. Some theoretical lenses involve ways of knowing and their relationship to affective literacy. For the purposes of this text, it is useful to differentiate curriculum content and pedagogy into different domains of knowing and contemporary curriculum models. It is becoming more obvious what might be involved in creating current domains for using or evaluating affective pedagogy. We could use approaches such as small groups, reflection methods, pictures, psychodrama, or even role play. We could also examine affective pedagogy by looking at how the student is learning—aesthetic, personal, ethical, or intersubjective. Another approach for assessing what is occurring related to affective pedagogy is to examine our affective methods by looking at contemporary educational theories such as social, critical pedagogy, learning community, and phenomenological landscape theories or a combination of these theories.

CHAPTER 2

Reviewing Traditional Teaching Methods

HISTORICAL TRADITIONAL TEACHING

Traditional teachers are those who typically send content and facts to their students and then hope the learner will understand the information. In addition, they test these students on how well they understand. Educators created this form of teaching through years of practice and now call it *traditional* classroom teaching. Some have called it an *instruction paradigm* in contrast to their desire to see more of a *learner paradigm* (Barr, 1998). Freire (1970/2009), a leading international educator of the 20th century, named this form of teaching a *banking teaching theory.*

> The teacher is no longer the only expert but instead is someone who joins with the student in the learning process. (Finke, 2009, p. 11)

> In the banking concept of education, knowledge is a gift bestowed by those who consider themselves knowledgeable upon those who they consider to know nothing. Projecting an absolute ignorance onto others. . . . (p. 72)

The banking method of teaching provides the student with *deposits* of knowledge like money in a bank. The process is teacher-focused and reinforces the power differential between teacher and student, which in turn encourages oppressive behaviors on the part of the student.

In many cases, nursing faculty want to see if students can perform, so the students are placed in a clinical lab to develop psychomotor skills or to integrate some experiential learning. There is a delicate balance created between skills that are specific for patient safety versus skills that the instructor demonstrates as ways to keep out variance or student creativity. The intent in the latter teaching method is to end up with complete conformity. When we examine how we conduct nursing foundations courses, we can see how well we meet this conformity model. Right or wrong, we often look for the expectation of conformity as a means to higher quality.

This trend toward conformity in education can be studied throughout higher education's history. American higher education started at Harvard in 1636, and the statement below outlines what higher education was originally like.

> Electives were unheard of, and all students (only males) were obliged to complete the same curriculum in lock-step fashion. Finally, antebellum colleges seem to have been prone to a peculiarly lifeless pedagogy, one consisting of little more than formal lectures, exercises in rote memorization, and formal disputation and recitation. (Lucas, 1996, p. 51)

It is easy to see that certain aspects of American higher education have not changed much in over 375 years. This lack of change may be problematic when it comes to pedagogy and the classroom. Have faculty become too accustomed and entrenched to this type of education? Or are they ready to explore something else? *Traditional teachers* focus pedagogy toward the needs of the instructor—not the needs of the student or of learning. It is convenient, easy, and thought to be more objective. Most teachers want it to stay this way. Traditional teachers forget there is a whole person attending their classes and this person may have even greater insights into patient needs than we are teaching. It appears that even those who want more experiential or affective learning have done little to make the change. It could be for a variety of reasons, but the fact is that much of nursing practice is exactly as it has been for over 40 years.

> The intuitive mind is a sacred gift and the rational mind is a faithful servant. We have created a society that honors the servant and has forgotten the gift. (Einstein, found in Secretan, 2004, p. 178)

Educational institutions have been criticized for decades for not being places of learning (Barr, 1998; Boyer, 1990; O'Brien, 1986; Wulff & Austin, 2004), and old debates have their own level of equilibrium. When debates become normalized and lose energy, there is no perception that a problem still exists. Has education really moved away from the 19th-century European educational model? Some have even argued that the instructional paradigm as defined by Barr should be continued, and many reject all educational imperatives that teachers have responsibilities for student learning or need for a learning paradigm. Boyer presented Gottinger's 1860 statement regarding faculty being specialists and not teachers: "He [the teacher] is not responsible for the success of his students. He is responsible only for the quality of his instruction. His duty begins and ends with himself" (Boyer, 1990, p. 120). In a world where we often hold to principles of self-accountability and self-responsibility, it is hard to consider anything other than what Gottinger stated in 1860.

Several researchers have suggested that quality instruction is the ability to teach students in a variety of ways in order to accommodate the different learning styles of the students (Mather & Champagne, 2008; Piane, Rydman, & Rudens, 1996; Vermunt & Vermetten, 2004; Wolfe, Bates, Manikowske, & Amundsen, 2006). This does not mean that teachers have moved away from a traditional teaching paradigm, but it could mean additional variations in teaching that are still cognitively focused. These same studies suggest that student programs of study seem to be an indicator for what their learning style will be. Engineering and education majors seem to prefer the traditional teaching model with their least favorite teaching method being an active self-regulating learning (Hativa & Birenbaum, 2000).

There are several additional factors that keep traditional teaching alive, including what some students want. Barr (1998) suggests that we continue to filter our desire to promote learning through the instructional paradigm by maintaining structures that support it. These are:

1. Having one teacher per course
2. Using one classroom
3. Not adjusting the classroom setting
4. Accepting the 50-minute class period
5. Conducting courses in 15- to 18-week blocks
6. Failing to provide opportunities for reflection and other affective pedagogy
7. Following curriculum designs that are not always focused on learning

Barr continues by stating, "I suppose the lecture is not defended as the ideal educational [learning] form, but I can tell you that it is vigorously defended nonetheless" (p. 20). As you read Vignette 2.1, ask yourself if this is your norm.

Vignette 2.1

Teacher: "Good morning class. We left off at slide 32, so we will pick up there."

The room is slightly dimmed as the PowerPoint slides are projected onto the screen. No more eye contact between student and teacher is possible while students open the printed handouts that have three slides per page on the left side of the page, and lines for taking notes on the right side of the page.

(continued)

Teacher: "Today you will learn about the three basic types of learning—cognitive, affective, and psychomotor. Let's look at their definitions."

The teacher's voice is heard in the dimly lit room, clarifying the definitions with a periodic question being asked after being prompted by the teacher who says, "Any questions?" The room is silent as students use various means to remember these definitions, for they will surely be on an examination at a later date. Some ignore all this one-way communication as they multitask by texting, surfing the Internet, or writing a note home to mom. After all, the definitions are on the slides, ready to be memorized at a later date.

Is the teaching described in Vignette 2.1 the norm you want and the one that is habitually played out in your classrooms? Or have you been looking for an alternative to the instructional teaching model?

Freire (1970/2009) suggests a deeper and often unconscious reason for keeping this traditional instructional teaching method alive. He states, "Education as the exercise of domination stimulates the credulity of students, with the ideological intent (often not perceived by educators) of indoctrinating them to adapt to the world of oppression" (p. 78). Could it be that we need everyone to know their place in society and that we run our schools and universities in such a way to keep people from revolting, or is it as simple as making the life of the instructor easier? Whatever keeps most educators teaching in this traditional or instructional mode is certainly powerful, as very little has changed in the approach for almost four centuries.

TRADITIONS IN NURSING EDUCATION

In keeping with the traditional instructional teaching model, nursing education continued to hear a loud voice from educators such as Lysaught (1970) who argued that such soft academic nursing education ought to be dropped in favor of more scientific and rationality-based education. He equated the nurturing side of nursing with being a feminine trait and thought it should be taken out of the training process. Prior to 1960, nursing education was primarily a hospital-based program that had demanding lectures that were integrated into many hours of practice and strict supervision. However, hospital-based nursing education was not seen as being *scientific,* and it was perceived to lack rational and objective thinking. Lysaught wanted to see that changed and for nursing to be more aligned with medicine.

Nursing education has been bombarded with the need to objectify all the various content that was being built around nursing taxonomies, nursing diagnoses, and nursing theory. Nearly 50 years ago, Krathwohl, Bloom, and Masia (1964) developed a learning taxonomy that focused on educational objectives in the affective domains of learning. These authors began their study by examining affective objectives in various college courses in the 1940s. Their findings indicated a continuous erosion of affective objectives as they watched the courses change over 10 and then 20 years. By 1964, Krathwohl et al. concluded that there was little, if any, attempt to include affective course objectives in curricula that had previously incorporated them.

During the same period as Lysaught's push for more objectivity, we started hearing from our first nursing theorists. King (1971), Orem (1971), Roger (1971), and Roy (1976) were presenting various ways to articulate nursing practice. However, not everyone was willing to call nursing a rational scientific practice. King stated, "Teachers who create a climate for learning help individuals see things in new ways, explore meaning, feelings, attitudes, and behavior of self and others, and understanding relationships between knowledge and its use in nursing practice" (p. 43). What a contrast to Lysaught (1970) who was looking for higher levels of rational technical approaches to reduce the subjective side of nursing.

Muddy Water

Other academic challenges preventing affective learning models have come from our historical reliance on rationalism and objectivity. From Plato to the turn of the 20th century, philosophers and educational leaders alike attempted to separate the intelligent, educated mind from the mind associated with experience and emotions. Physicians also wanted to eliminate the idea that they were *empirical,* as this would imply they were using trial-and-error strategies for practice and were therefore lacking in *scientific training* (Dewey, 1916/1944, p. 264) to guide their practice. (Note that the definition of empirical had a different meaning in 1916 and was called a trial-and-error approach by Dewey in contrast to a scientific approach.) The push was for pure reason and Kantian objectivity to guide the professional of the time and to control for researcher bias. It is also important to note that Immanuel Kant (1724–1804) was a German philosopher using Descartes's rationalism and Locke's empiricism as he refuted inductive reasoning as not valid, and then used highly complex thinking regarding how we observe things. However, he was the first to acknowledge that "some of the properties observed in objects may be due to the nature of the observer rather than the objects themselves" (Flew, 1984, p. 190).

At the same time, a mixed message was being sent regarding reality. Clinicians also integrated "pure reason thinking and Spirit as something morally praiseworthy" (Dewey, 1916/1944, p. 265). There continued to be distinctions drawn between absolute truths in the external-objective world versus what became internalized as a subjective state or a spiritual world, which was viewed as metaphysical science.

Emotions have often been perceived to be purely private and personal, having nothing to do with the work of pure intelligence, as a result of early leaders in education such as Dewey. "The intellect is a pure light;

the emotions a disturbing heat" (Dewey, 1944/1916, p. 335). At the same time, Dewey was adamant that all education is a moral concern for the building of character, which would tie in with current definitions of affective development. It appears that his main aversion was focused specifically on emotions and their role in education. Needless to say, there was an early movement to embrace objectivism and reject that which was more subjective within education.

Tyler (1949) is credited with the idea that course objectives are needed for the purpose of measuring what is being taught. Does this sound familiar?: *The student will be able to describe the use of learning objectives in curriculum development.* Nursing faculty continue to live by this thinking. However, what some saw as important nursing teaching methods actually misrepresented the intent of the original author. Tyler states, "Education is a process of changing the behavioral patterns of people. This is using behavior in the broad sense to include *thinking* and *feeling* as well as overt actions" (pp. 5–6). His work included "generalized patterns of behavior" (p. 46) that were not only objectively measurable verbs as we use today, but also included subjective statements. One example Tyler provides is "to develop social attitudes" (p. 46). Given the tendency toward objectivity in nursing education, imagine the response from state boards of nursing or credentialing agencies as they review syllabi and find subjective goals are being used for the course outcomes. Faculty might consider running out the door as the credentialing agencies read anything but objective adjectives that can be measured using empirical methods. It might be a good time to ask, "How did we ever get this far into objectivity?"

This era was full of push and pull by those thinking about what was needed but who found the academic environment ill-prepared to deal with so much subjective thinking. In the limited classes where affective pedagogy was being provided, there was little knowledge of how it was being implemented and how affective education might be improved. This continuous distrust of the subjective and an affective experience that involves emotions in the classroom, permeated this entire era and in many ways continues to be an academic struggle. The recent study by Benner, Sutphen, Leonard, and Day (2010) brings us right back to the conflict:

> Experiential learning is one of the strengths of nursing education; we found a sharp contrast between the classroom situation, where it was the most absent, and the clinical situations, where it is common. . . . Although we applaud the exceptions to this finding, classroom teachers who make an effort to integrate the classroom and clinical experiences, and the even fewer who make the classroom a setting for rich, experiential learning. (pp. 64–65)

These authors do not articulate *affective teaching* methods but describe their experiential learning methods as affective methods that impact the students more deeply and personally, and how they impact their knowing who they are becoming.

According to Smith-Coletta, the former editor of *Nurse Educator* and the *Journal of Nursing Administration*, "Educators have the responsibility and obligation to bring values, attitudes, feelings, and beliefs into conscious awareness" (King, 1984, p. x). This type of pedagogy was not seen as easy and demanded that academia change its views of teaching and learning—but would they? Elizabeth King wrote the first book on *Affective Education in Nursing* in 1984. It was not considered a theory, but rather a method of teaching that centered on values clarification, moral development, and problem solving. Her work could easily be viewed today as advocating cultural awareness that includes a host of experiential classroom methods. King's (1984) methods incorporated:

- Group discussion to include how the instructor should interact with the students
- Case study method that included moral and behavioral dilemmas
- Role play that was given measurement tools
- Simulation gaming that included pros and cons for its use

King was also involved in the objectivist movement, as were most educators of the time. She continued to identify learning objectives in their most traditional sense—staying free of the subjective side of affective pedagogy. However, that would not preclude a student from having a deep growth response from these methods. What is amazing is that King's book in complete form was rarely available in any academic setting, and in 35 years of practice and nursing education I've never seen her book used.

Being tossed from one spectrum of nursing education to the opposite is a time of muddy water in our academic history. It seems to have also been true for all higher education. In an example of how challenging the muddy water can be for faculty, Vignette 2.2 provides a bit of humor regarding an instructor who thinks it is time to bring some affective pedagogy into his or her teaching, but wants to do so in the same way the instructor normally does everything.

Vignette 2.2

Joan is my staff assistant and has been very helpful when I am rushed and struggling to get caught up. I have recently heard about various ways of improving my classroom, so I enlist Joan's assistance. "Joan, would you go to the university bookstore for me, and go to the affective teaching section of the store. I need two printed, paper pads of student acknowledgment and recognition sheets, a thimble of personal self-disclosure with some good examples, a classroom discussion stimulator, two posters on student follow-up reminders, one flexibility integrator, a book on acceptance of feelings in

(continued)

classrooms, and a tape recorder that is automatically programmed for timely feedback that has a 'being present' button on it.

"Also, pick up one 16-gig care pedagogy faculty chip that allows vocal expressiveness and smiling, and includes an eye contact and relaxed body posture setting. It needs to be the 'CARE 4U' chip that uses active listening digital capability.

"Just tell the store to bill it to my department here at the college. Thanks for doing this for me. I have to get my slide presentation ready for class so I appreciate your help. Oh, one more thing. Bring me a can of My Way energy drink. Thanks."

SUMMARY

It is clear that our American educational system was born from a desire to maintain an objective method of teaching in the cognitive domain of learning. Faculty carried the information, which was then passed on to their students, and this cognitive information was *banked*, to be recalled at a later time. This is called an *institutional paradigm* or *traditional teaching* in this text as a means of distinguishing it from a *learning-centered* teaching approach. This historical foundation allows us to take this journey to examine the need to integrate the subjective domain of knowing, called affective teaching, which brings values, attitudes, feelings, and beliefs into conscious awareness for students during their learning process. There were early attempts to be more holistic, relational, and even subjectively focused, but with poor results. There was fear and a distrust of the subjective, a dedication and commitment to the rational objective where Kantianism was the philosophy of the day, and an incorrect interpretation of Tylerian objectivism as pure objectivism for purposes of measurement.

King (1971) was already asking nursing instructors to become relational educators and to look for intersubjective knowing as she presented her theory of nursing practice. As she states, "The teacher of nursing practice guides the learner as both grow and mature in the process of teaching and learning" (p. 43). Or, as noted by Watson (1985, p. 59), "We learn from one another how to be more human by identifying ourselves with others and finding their dilemmas in ourselves. What we all learn from it is self-knowledge."

CHAPTER 3

Planting the Objectivist Movement in Nursing Education

As discussed in Chapter 2, except for a small minority of leaders who have focused on care theory, nursing education and professional organizations have generally been pushing to be more objective. In the broader community of higher education, we have seen the same movement. A small voice continues to be heard by such educators as Parker Palmer and Nel Nodding. Palmer (2007) put it this way:

> Teaching, like any truly human activity, emerges from one's inwardness for better or worse. As I teach, I project the condition of my soul onto my students, my subject, and our way of being together. The entanglements I experience in the classroom are often no more or less than the convolutions of my inner life. Viewed from this angle, teaching holds a mirror to the soul. (pp. 2–3)

> Objectivism set out to put truth on firmer ground than the whims of princes and priests, and for that we can be grateful. But history is full of ironies, and one of them is the way objectivism has bred new versions of the same evils it tried to correct. (Palmer, 2007, p. 53)

Just imagine how subjective the idea of looking at one's inner soul would be. It is not a mathematical formula, but a complex integration of physiology, anatomy, chemistry, electricity, microorganisms, mind, psychology, and a life force that many associate with his or her creator. How much of this is really objective? How much of what we present in the classroom is really objective versus subjective information? Don't judge it, but consider the reality of this fully human phenomenon.

Wilber (2000) suggests that we have three realities asking to be heard and integrated. The first is the *subjective truth*, the second is the *objective truth,* and the third is the *intersubjective truth.* "It is toward just such an integral model that we can now turn" (p. 73). Intersubjective truth is a very complicated subject that needs additional discussion, as we look at how quantum mechanics (physics) impacts us personally, which includes our teaching.

SCIENCE OF THE SUBJECTIVE

The period from 1980 to 2000 was filled with proposed strategies to include subjective reality—the affective domain—and has started to bring a sense of approval for the science of the subjective. During this era, more was occurring than simply pedagogy experimentation in nursing, education, and science. There was a growth of qualitative research projects by faculty and doctoral students; however, their studies continued to be called *soft science* and were placed on the lower levels of the research evidence pyramids (Burns & Grove, 2008).

Additionally, science was starting to receive significant challenges as to what it means to be *scientific.* The Princeton Engineering Anomalies Research (PEAR) Center (www.princeton.edu/~pear) has been conducting quantum research for years with some significant results. PEAR researchers have conducted hundreds of experiments on the mysteries of quantum physics to include human consciousness studies. Jahn and Dunne (1997) acknowledged the debate regarding objective and subjective science and suggest that both must be used to have a real understanding of what may be occurring in the real world in which we are engaged. They state:

> The thesis is thus that science must soon make a deliberate and considered choice whether to continue to deny all subjective currency access to its table of scholarly business, thus excluding itself from comprehension of the universe of aesthetics and creative experience, including that which bears on objective effects, or to broaden its purview to encompass these softer parameters in some disciplined yet productive fashion. (p. 207)

There is a need to see the subjective domain as legitimate and capable of being studied in a way that gives new knowledge and understanding. "All told, some 50 million experimental trials have been performed to this date, containing more than 3 billion bits of binary information" (Jahn & Dunn, 1997, p. 209). These 50 million experimental trials show evidence of links between the subjective human experience and how they can impact our world in consistently measurable ways that are not just random outcomes. When the subjective quantum and conscious intention experiments are totaled, the results are impressive: "The composite anomaly is unlikely by chance to be less than one part in a trillion" (p. 209), or $P < 0.000000000001$ for those statisticians who enjoy P values. All these studies lead to this result, "It seems inescapable to conclude that operator consciousness is capable of inserting information, in its most rudimentary *objective* form of binary bits, into these random physical systems, by some anomalous means that is independent of space and time" (pp. 210–211). In other words, our thoughts can influence the physical world and we can never be truly separated from that which we are studying. You can blind or double-blind but not really prevent this impact on the object under study. The act of observation in itself impacts what we are studying. This is a challenging thought for all the objectivists that believe we need to be more objective in our science, in our classrooms, in our testing, and in our pedagogical strategies. Imagine if all such thought is just an illusion to make us feel better about what we are doing—sticking to our objectivist rationalism.

Unfortunately, a meta-synthesis as described by Jahn and Dunne did not seem to impact the academic thinking in any significant way during this period or even today. We continue to want more objectivity, and therefore we associate being educated with using scientific thinking and positivistic thinking that emphasize quantitative research methods and deductive reasoning. It seems like heresy to think otherwise. Palmer (2007) suggests a different perspective on objectivism:

> Objectivism, far from telling the truth about how we know, is a myth meant to feed our fading fantasy of science, technology, power, and control. If we dare to move through our fear, to practice knowing as a form of love, we might abandon our illusion of control and enter a partnership with the otherness [students] of the world. (p. 57)

Subjective reality, which encompasses the affective domain of teaching, is in direct contrast to the objectivist and rationalist movement that surrounded the philosophies that were expressed through such authors as Ayn Rand in the 1970s and 1980s (http://www.youtube.com/watch?v=1ooKsv_SX4Y&feature=youtu.be and http://www.youtube.com/watch?v=4doTzCs9lEc&feature=youtu.be). The objectivist movement was designed to separate spirituality from science, or faith from reality, and its proponents believed that only objectivism was capable of finding reality in our world. It is said that Rand's work was seen by a host of secularists, educators, and entire institutions as a way to be more accurate with universal truths and that it supported the movement to separate what was believed to be the inferior subjective universe, including issues of faith and God, from the scientific and so-called truth-giving objective universe.

Nursing leadership, nursing state boards, and certification boards continue to ask nurses to update their knowledge. In the process of updating their continuing education, there is the expectation of having objective learning outcomes for all such training, but inner awareness, maturational growth, or subjectivity are usually not required. Benner, Sutphen, Leonard, and Day (2010) state:

> At this point, nurses are left to their own self-assessment and selection of continuing education from a range of continuing education classes. Although most health care organizations have become centers of teaching and learning in their own right, they focus mainly on teaching new technologies and new regulations, both of which are necessary but do not offer the clinical knowledge and skilled know-how needed for a self-improving practice. (p. 19)

This push toward objectively measurable nursing outcomes in continuing education further emphasizes a separation between subjectivity and objectivity and plays into our thinking about what it means to be an educated person or nurse.

During an age of mandatory separation, many, including Pearson (1911/2007) in his work *The Grammar of Science,* pushed the need to separate all subjective thinking from scientific inquiry in order to be an educated and credible person. Even to this day, faculty courses and evaluations do not address their affective teaching methods or outcomes (Ornstein, 1995). Ornstein states:

> Depending on the instrument or checklist utilized, a teacher might be judged "good" or "effective" by coming to class on time, writing clear objectives on the blackboard, monitoring seatwork, or reviewing homework—criteria that overlook the emotional and human qualities of teaching the real "stuff" that is at the heart of teaching. Evaluation instruments tend to favor teachers adept in behaviorist tasks or teaching facts and skills, partly because the instruments focused on small segments of observable or measurable teacher behaviors, and because the tests that measured student outcomes were knowledge based. (p. 124)

Ornstein references Craig and Eisner to support his belief that faculty will "face subtle discrimination" as they attempt to stress "the abstract, divergent thinking, humanistic or moral practices, . . . and hard-to-measure processes" (p. 124).

Although there may be professional risks to incorporating the affective domain, as presented in Chapter 1, today we are learning that reforming education necessitates evaluation of the value of subjectivity in our teaching methods. The push against pure objectivism is a theme for international reformers of education such as Paulo Freire who wrote a book to teachers in 1998 and stated, "It is impossible to teach without the courage to love, without the courage to try a thousand times before giving in. In short, it is impossible to teach without a forged, invented, and well-thought-out capacity to love" (p. 42). Darder (2002) presents an entire book, *Reinventing Paulo Freire: A Pedagogy of Love*, and offers a strong reminder of how love is the pedagogy of relationships, intersubjective knowing, and being present for students. We are in a struggle, or even a battle of sorts. Even if our academic mentors and professional organizations want us to accept the various ways of knowing, the push is for us to only accept one form as true knowing—the empirical or objective form. Palmer (2007) believes the abandonment of the subjective has very serious ramifications for our students, and states:

> "[The] self-protective" split of personhood from practice is encouraged by an academic culture that distrusts personal truth. Though the academy claims to value multiple modes of knowing, it honors only one—an "objective" way of knowing that takes us into the "real" world by taking us "out of ourselves." . . . The academic bias against subjectivity not only forces our students to write poorly ("it is believed . . ." instead of "I believe . . . ") but also deforms their thinking about themselves and their world. In a single stroke, we delude our students into thinking that bad prose can turn opinions into facts, and we alienate them from their own inner lives. (pp. 18–19)

Fear of the subjective has created serious flaws in our academic system and in the thinking of our students. In nursing, the work of Lysaught (1970) pushed nursing educators to question the *caring practices* as moving nursing away from "the technical and instrumental work of nurses" (Benner, Sutphen, Leonard, & Day, 2010, p. 23). It did not stop there. As nursing theorists were developing their ideas of what nursing is, most did not articulate *caring* as a major construct of the profession. Fawcett (1995) presents the arguments from both sides, but ends up excluding *caring* as a major construct of what is unique to nursing. She believed a major construct (metaparadigm) must be "perspective-neutral" (p. 11). Again, nursing needed to keep things objective and free from value-laden possibilities; the profession was building its theoretical beliefs at the expense of really owning its caring practices. This was the positivist philosophy that then was used to guide the so-called "real scientific research" we call quantitative research. The more we could control the extraneous variables, the better the research.

So the question is this: Which type of nurses do you want to treat you? Which type of nurses do you want teaching the next generation of nurses? Should nursing be devoid of caring theory as a core practice found in our foundation courses, or should it be as high an expectation as getting vital signs correctly? If we provide the knowledge for our nursing students to be technically competent, will we have an equal expectation that they are compassionate, empathetic, and able to form relationships with their patients? Vignette 3.1 provides an example of how the latter might be practiced in a foundations course.

Vignette 3.1

At the beginning of your shift, when you are meeting your new patient, start with this partnering exercise. (It actually takes approximately 3 minutes unless you do the assessment or pain management during this time).

1. Tell the patient your name and your role as you sit at eye level.
2. Ask the patient his or her priorities for the day, so you can assist him or her in meeting these goals.
3. Let the patient know what your practice needs are during your shift and look at integrating your needs and the patient's needs for the day.
4. Put your name, contact number, and partnered goals on the white board in the room.
5. Continue with the Five Ps:
   a. You did Partnering already
   b. Ask about restroom needs—Potty
   c. Obtain a Pain assessment
   d. Make Positioning adjustments
   e. Check the Pump to reduce potential noise distractions
6. Address pain or your first assessment of the day and do both soon.
7. Before leaving, ask if there is anything he or she needs before you return after your regular rounds to provide additional care.

THE IMPACT OF QUANTUM MECHANICS

As discussed in regard to research by Jahn and Dunne (1997), one of the most powerful ways of connecting the objective and subjective realms is to examine recent work in quantum mechanics. The current resurgence of quantum mechanics is quite clear in its premise of stating that the observer is never able to separate from that which he or she observes (Rosenblum & Kuttner, 2006). Quantum mechanics suggests we will always tamper with the object in some way simply by our observation as we assess or measure the research subject. Even Plato asked the question, "Is the physical world shaped in some sense by our perceptions of it?" (Horgan, 1992, p. 1). The advent of quantum mechanics has and will continue to leave its mark on what we now believe to be real, that is, knowing the process of observation without intrusion impacts the observed in significant ways.

> An unobserved quantum entity is said to exist in a *coherent superposition* of all the possible *states* permitted by its *wave function*. But as soon as an observer makes a measurement capable of distinguishing between these states, the wave function collapses, and the entity is forced into a single state. (Horgan, 1992, p. 4)

You may be thinking that it will be necessary to ignore quantum mechanics in your view of the world and scientific inquiry. There are good reasons why you might think this way; even Einstein shrank from it because it challenged his sense of reality.

> Quantum mechanics conflicts violently not only with our intuition but perhaps even with the scientific worldview we have held since the 1600s. Nevertheless, because quantum theory satisfies Galileo's criterion—that of experimental verification—physicists readily accept it as the underlying basis of all physics and thus of all science. (Rosenblum & Kuttner, 2006, p. 23)

There are some key principles to quantum mechanics that we will return to, but needless to say, it challenges the objectivist view with the best science we know.

In the 1970s, an anesthesiologist who had been integrating quantum mechanics into his practice stated something that has shaken me since I first read it. "Doctors and social scientists remain the most adamant and still the greatest exponents of so-called objective studies based on 'empirical' data. The fact is that there is no such thing as objective science in our day" (Yanovasky, 1978, p. 113). More recently, a physician and professor of medicine at the University of California at Los Angeles stated, "Objectivity can make you blind" (Remen, 1999, p. 47). Do you think we can be objective observers? Can you continue to accept the form of thinking that states a person is being objective about a decision by using blinded or double-blinded studies?

Perhaps there must also be an intersubjective reality as presented by Ken Wilber and reinforced by quantum mechanics, because when we observe a phenomenon we ask it to form a singular place in space. Prior to our observing it, it has the potential to be in many places, or it can even be energy versus matter.

McFarlane (1995) takes the ideas of quantum mechanics even further and integrates the ideas of the first quantum researchers and theorists, Werner Heisenberg and Niels Bohr—both pioneer physicists of the 20th century. McFarlane states:

> These people make the outrageous claim that we normally live in the delusion that there is a real objective world. Since this seems to be a blatant contradiction with both our immediate experience and everything most of us were ever taught, our natural response is to dismiss it as ludicrous. . . . If we are to be honest with ourselves, we had better think twice before dismissing what Bohr and Heisenberg have to say and take a closer look. (p. 2)

Two video clips may offer you more than you ever wanted to know about quantum mechanics. However, it is helpful to watch both of them. To ignore what they say means you are willing to stay in the illusion of thinking you know what is real and objective, or not. You may not want to stay in that place.

The history of how Bohr's and Heisenberg's theories finally came together is illustrated at http://www.youtube.com/watch?v=45KGS1Ro-sc&feature=youtu.be and http://www.youtube.com/watch?v=7u_UQG1La1o&feature=youtu.be offers a simplified example of what was really discovered and its impact on what we observe in this universe. Quantum mechanics makes several powerful claims that have never been disproved, and is the science of our time that encompasses all scientific thinking (Rosenblum & Kuttner, 2006). We just don't like to discuss it, as it seems illogical to think that "reality is not fixed, but fluid, or mutable, and hence possibly open to influences" (McTaggart, 2007, p. xx). That does not mean it can be ignored for the sake of objective research methods that we hold to so dearly. If nursing is to be a research-based profession, we must consider what is our best science and how it impacts us as nurses. It is one thesis that quantum mechanics actually helps us integrate the subjective practices we believe in as real science, and this includes spirituality, healing presence, caring presence, the influences of prayer, and relational-centered healing.

The value in studying quantum mechanics is that it enables us to easily see that the world is not always as it seems and that subjectivity has a role to play in determining any outcome. For example, a quantum mechanics clip (found at http://www.youtube.com/watch?v=v0v-cvvyc-M&feature=youtu.be) discusses multiple positioning, entanglement, and the "double slit," or Young experiments, which will certainly challenge the reality of objectivity and inquiry controls for any researcher. Clips from *What the Bleep Do We Know: Down the Rabbit Hole* (2004), and the text on this subject (Arntz, Chasse, & Vicente, 2005), take everything we thought of as real and place it in the world of an illusion that we create just to make us feel better about what we believe. However, we must learn to live in this world and create a healthy respect for the real science of our day—quantum mechanics.

The double slit experiments prove that particles can turn to energy waves, or stay particles if there is an observer. Particles have the potential to be energy or matter depending on whether they are observed or not (see en.wikipedia.org/wiki/Double-slit_experiment). Silverman (2010) wrote a book dedicated to these quantum mind-bending concepts and discusses the idea that superposition particles or waves can be in thousands of locations at the very same time unless someone observes them. Then they move into a singular position so we can all see the same thing. Where is the objectivity in that?

One might expect that Martha Rogers has a very different view of nursing, as she introduced nursing to the world of quantum mechanics. However, she struggled to use and integrate this new science, as the science itself was still evolving. Statements such as "people are inseparable from the natural world" (Rogers, 1970, p. 49) and her statement that "man and environment are continuously exchanging matter and energy with one another" (p. 54) indicate her use of quantum mechanics in its infancy. However, she too was a theorist looking for objectivity and provided scientific verification of what nurses were up to in her text, leaving us to wonder how much of quantum mechanics she was willing to integrate.

Recognizing that the complexities of quantum mechanics may prove challenging to understand does not require you to be an expert in quantum mechanics, but it does raise the realization that there is something seriously flawed in our thinking when we have a need to create higher levels of objectivity as a way to find the best truth. It is important to remember, "Objectivity can make you blind" (Remen, 1999, p. 47).

A NEW RESEARCH PARADIGM

Given the previous discussions of traditional research methods that have been used to study affective teaching and now the introduction of quantum mechanics, you may wonder how you might advance the study of affective teaching methods using the most recent physics and philosophy at our disposal. But you shouldn't worry about balancing the two. It is true that when educators use this different lens to examine their thinking regarding reality, inquiry, and teaching, they will also need to refine their research and assessment tools. But one would fail if attempting to examine gravity by using something other than Newtonian physics. The same is true when examining the subjective. It is critical to use the proper philosophy and inquiry methods for such a unique domain, and it may be the reason so many historical authors have struggled with the notion of measuring, assessing, or conducting research on the subjective experience.

It may be just as true that we cannot separate the objective from the subjective in our need to measure or investigate results. It may be time that the traditional methods of assessing various forms of research be reconstructed to an *integral* methodology where we would expect to see more use of triangulation, cross-over designs, action research, and constructivism. There is an obvious failing when we attempt to use the traditional core methods of research such as experimental designs that demand a control group, intervention, and randomization. Such an approach expects us to think as positivists and that we can control our world in various ways to be more objective using deductive methods.

Likert (1932) was one of the first researchers to be concerned with the idea of being able to measure the subjective concept of social attitudes, which were thought to be endless in possibilities or even impossible to objectively measure. His historic work has led to many strategies where the subjective number scales have been refined, revised, and have sometimes given rise to false statistical methods. Likert states:

> On this basis one of our cardinal problems is to find whether social attitudes, in this sense, can be shown to be measurable, and if an affirmative answer is forthcoming, a serious attempt must be made to justify the separation of one attitude from others. (p. 8)

The very first Likert scale testing was specifically designed to examine a "'judgment of value' rather than a 'judgment of fact'" (p. 12). The objectification of the subjective experience is not new, but many foundational principles of reality have changed since the turn of the 20th century.

Interpretive Inquiry

Additional challenges are related to states of truth and their relationship to objectivity and subjectivity as discussed earlier. Some have argued that neither alone is truth. "Reality resides neither with an objective external world nor with the subjective mind of the person knowing, but within dynamic transactions between the two" (Barone, 1992, p. 31). Rogers also argued that we cannot dichotomize the objective from the subjective and suggested that everything is actually connected—supporting quantum mechanics. One of her postulates states, "Man is a unified whole possessing his own integrity and manifesting characteristics that are more than and different from the sum of his parts" (Rogers, 1970, p. 47).

There are many who have or will begin to question the scientific rigor when there is an integration of the subjective to make an objective observation or measurement more valid. I believe that the objective and subjective must work together for the best knowledge to be identified. This integration seems to violate the positivist philosophy of a singular reality that can be found by the deductive process of dissecting something into its smallest and measurable parts in order to obtain the best truth. Such thinking is certainly not acceptable, as integrative thinkers look at subjective experiences that impact the individual's affective development related to feelings, values, ethics, and a sense of the self or who one is becoming.

There appeared to be a growing swell by contemporary higher education researchers and theorists from the mid-1980s to the mid-1990s who articulated a need for a new research paradigm that included the use of qualitative methods and alternative philosophies of inquiry (Conrad, 1989; Heshusius, 1994; Leslie & Beckham, 1986; Lincoln & Guba, 1985; Ornstein, 1995; Peterson, 1986). For example, Lincoln and Guba's (1985) classic work highlighted the need for researchers of human experience to consider ethical issues related to the continued use of the positivistic attitudes regarding inquiry. They argued effectively that naturalistic methods are more appropriate for human experience studies. Ornstein (1995) encouraged the use of narrative research that used thick or qualitatively rich descriptions instead of statistical inference when one researches teaching methods. Could it be that there is a need for an interpretive inquiry method to assess affective teaching, allowing the investigator to observe and be a part of that dynamic while seeking understanding as to what transpired in the classroom between faculty and students?

The historical literature describes various methods of interpreting human experiences. Polkinghorne (1983) discussed hermeneutic systems and phenomenology as a developing movement, including the work of Dilthey, Husserl, Heidegger, Merleau-Ponty, Gadamer, Ricoeur, Shultz, Weber, and Habermas. This movement focused on "human experience as it is lived"

(Polkinghorne, p. 201) and involves accessing the meaning of action and not just the presence of action. Interpreting meaningful action originated with the Greek word *hermeneuein,* which means to interpret. Not all hermeneutic theorists, as listed by Polkinghorne, agree on what it means to have a hermeneutic study, and it is more useful to move to an eclectic term of *interpretive inquiry* to describe the interpretation of affective pedagogy.

Interpretive inquiry requires rigorous examination of a large body of data. When conducting an interpretive inquiry, the researcher takes great care to meet certain scientific rigors that are designed to validate the data. One such rigor may be to triangulate the data, which means that connection and correlation are made from two or more data sources or perspectives that may include objective and subjective data (Burns & Grove, 2008; Glesne & Peshkin, 1992). As a starting point for studying affective teaching, a triangulated approach seems to be an excellent beginning. There are increasing methodological challenges, however, to taking a triangulated approach. Consider when an ethnographer is sitting on the urban streets trying to take in an entire interactive, dynamic city street in New York, or a classroom researcher is sitting day after day in a class examining a classroom from various perspectives. Richardson (1994) called this comprehensive data integration *crystallization* and stated, "Crystallization provides us with a deepened, complex, thoroughly partial understanding of the topic. Paradoxically, we know more and doubt what we know" (p. 522). Crystallization occurs when data come from multiple points and then are collectively seen as a theme, or when a theme emerges from the data. Greene (1994) clearly articulated the paradoxical tension experienced by the interpretivist inquirer: "On one hand, interpretivist evaluators need methodological quality assurances for their audiences. On the other hand, the very idea of prescriptions for quality or any other methodological concern is philosophically inconsistent with the basic tenets of interpretivism" (p. 37).

This chapters identifies several philosophical shifts that would make meaningless a statement that suggests we cannot measure the subjective, such as affective teaching methods. Not only can we evaluate the objective actions and practices seen, but we can also integrate this with the subjective experience in order to understand more of what has occurred. Thus, not only can we observe a phenomenon occurring, we can begin to ask questions regarding the motives of the participants in that phenomenon. This approach integrates objective observations with the subjective elements that influence an outcome for enhanced understanding overall. In addition, we look at the various phenomena in order to have deeper understanding of what was observed—called interpretive inquiry, or *hermeneutic research.*

The value of affective teaching is based on the subjective learning experiences of the student who has an inner experience that academics usually ignore in our assessments of the courses. Historically we have attempted to make everything measured in nursing more objective so we can be more assured that we can measure it. The research on intention experiments, consciousness experiments, and the reality of quantum mechanics suggest all this focus on objectivism is for naught. Objectivity is really an illusion we construct to make us feel better about what we are doing—able to measure with numbers, tools, and unbiased tampering. However, if we use methods, such as interpretive inquiry, we will be able to measure the subjective and objective as integrations of data that will give us our best understanding of what is happening. In addition, it does not require us to ignore key aesthetic and subjective nursing practices that center on caring or presence for fear we cannot measure it.

> We do not see things as they are. We see them as we are. A belief is like a pair of sunglasses. When we wear a belief and look at life through it, it is difficult to convince ourselves what we see is not what is real. (Remen, 1996, p. 77)

SUMMARY

During the period 1970 to 1990, extraordinary theories and philosophies by educators and scientists asked the academic world to be more accepting of the power of the subjective. These same educators and scientists also suggested there is a serious risk in ignoring this domain. The most significant risk for those rejecting the subjective is that one's objectivity is really an illusion rather than a closer approximation of reality and truth—it becomes a small adoration on our path to truth.

> Any search for new knowledge begins with some form of subjective experience, which consciousness then attempts to describe, catalogue, and comprehend by comparison with other previously catalogued and comprehended descriptions of experience. The metaphoric ladder thus constructed may reach lofty intellectual heights, but its lowest rungs inevitably rest on very subjective, perhaps even archetypal ground. (Jahn & Dunne, 1997, p. 217)

There is hope for educators and researchers who want to expand their knowledge of affective education or other subjective experiences. Valuing the subjective and integrating this with objective information helps us find additional knowledge that supports our understanding of this form of teaching. Quantum mechanics helps us have a healthy respect for an integrative approach that is best termed integrative inquiry, using crystallization as a way to interpret its multifaceted data to create meaning.

This chapter contains information that may shake the reader's sense of stability and his or her previous trust in the objective methods currently in place for guiding nursing practice and education. Go down this rabbit hole only as far as you feel safe. We will return to the ideas and principles that stem from these constructs as we progress in this text. As we move into the intersubjective truths, we will uncover more value and use of the principles stated here. This will give us a place to explore the idea that educators can partner with students in a way in which they know they are learners and teachers at the same time. Understanding the subjective at this level will offer us a greater chance of using this knowledge for such a purpose—and a sense of *love* will also be present. This awareness would give teachers a new sense of using *care pedagogy* and what they might be capable of when presenting affective teaching methods for their students. Vignette 3.2 is an example of bringing quantum mechanics and affective methods to the classroom.

Vignette 3.2

As I get ready to teach my next class, I read these lines to prepare my thinking: "When crossing a river, remove your sandals. When crossing a border, remove your crown" (White Hmong Proverb). As I walk to the classroom, I touch the door jamb, which is an action or ritual I have chosen to remind me that I have crossed the border to sacred ground. This is a place where the students and I will partner in our entanglement of knowing—an intersubjective knowing that will be knowledge building and insightful knowing for all of us.

I step away from the PowerPoint, the podium barrier, and expose my whole body as I speak of the blunt aggressive language a psychotic patient used with me in my past—and I know the aggressive tone was for his sense of safety and had nothing to do with me. As a new nurse, I was not certain it wasn't an attack on me, so I went off to recalibrate my own energy before returning to the unit. I was able to return, and provided an example to the students of how I valued the patient's needs and my own as I gave him space, time, no shame, and no personal projections related to my own vulnerability. I asked him if he could take his medication now, and I would check on him later as I stayed connected to him with a quiet tone, in a pleasant voice, and in a nonthreatening way.

The students are not sure they can do this as they start their mental health clinical rotations next week. I asked them to pair up, to look at each other, but give each other space. One is to talk about something he or she finds exciting and the other is to stay present and connect primarily nonverbally. They can ask a question, but they are not to use the word, "why." Two minutes is a long time to stay attentive. Now they need to discuss what that felt like for those 2 minutes. Many types of reactions were felt, and I wanted to hear if the one talking felt heard. If not, what caused the distraction? If yes, how did he or she believe the other student's therapeutic-self showed?

I ask the students to own their therapeutic-self, and to get to know it better. I ask them to be honest with any discomfort they may be feeling, and be willing to say what it is. And, I ask them to avoid words that generate a defensive response in others (e.g., the word "why"). They can write down these personal insights in their reflection books and digest what they have learned about themselves. I also jot down some notes about what I am learning just before I prepare for the next topic.

It is time to release fear of the subjective, to embrace it and bring quantum mechanics into the nursing profession with the use of intention and rituals. This will free us to think differently, which would include how to conduct research on teaching in new ways.

PART II

Affective Concepts, Strategies, and Methods

You cannot solve the problems of today with the same thinking that caused them.—Albert Einstein

CHAPTER 4

Building an Infrastructure for Affective-Literate Teachers

As we look at what is going on in many classrooms, we may be satisfied with what we see. Maybe we are teaching and suddenly think about the need to make the content more impactful by adding some new form of affective teaching method. Some may pull something out of their tool box of pedagogical strategies without realizing what it is they are really doing, and it just works. There are many levels of affective teaching, and some are certainly more risky than others. Research (Ondrejka, 1998) has taught us that faculty who are considered excellent teachers provide a variety of affective teaching methods, but they rarely have language to describe what it is they are doing.

> I suggest that if we want to free ourselves from objectivity, we need to fundamentally reorder our understanding of the relationship between self and other, and turn toward a participatory mode of consciousness. (Heshusius, 1994, p. 15)

CLASSROOM CULTURE PROMOTED BY CARE PEDAGOGY

Affective theories and practices have been used within the care paradigm of practice extensively in the 1990s and into the early 21st century. Several nursing authors have provided information on how care is viewed and used (Bevis & Watson, 1989; Gaut, 1992; Harrison, 1995; Hughes, 1995; Leininger & Watson, 1990; Schoenly, 1994; and Woods, 1993). All have suggested that teaching practices that encompass affective education are essential within nursing practice. Most of these authors define the affective domain as the *art of nursing.* They discuss affective literacy in the context of morals and values education using a host of strategies in keeping with the focus of the first nursing text on affective teaching by King (1984). King recommended the use of several affective methods of teaching in classrooms, which were discussed earlier:

1. Group discussion
2. Case studies
3. Role playing
4. Simulation gaming

Harrison (1995) also supported the idea of understanding through caring and the ethical knowing domain, while advocating the personal knowing of self as a primary tool to be used in nursing education.

Bevis and Watson (1989) suggested that the educator's challenge is complex, and that meaningful changes require changes in faculty attitudes. Faculty set the stage for defining the classroom culture, and it is faculty who make choices on shaping that culture. Bevis and Watson describe how faculty members need to foster a more affectively appropriate classroom by supporting:

> . . . [p]ermission giving, practice, and group approval for the normal warmth, concern, caring, and moral rectitude that characterize most nursing teachers. A climate of validation of self-worth; of wholeness; of perfect person; of good intent; of respect for one's needs, integrity, life choices, [life] styles; and personal and professional values is created in agreement and effort together. (p. 176)

Bevis and Watson present arguments and discussions regarding the care curriculum that include a paradigm shift in learning typology, teacher–student shifts with a focus on relationship building, and holistic, educative instruction. The concept of care goes beyond empathy and has a goal of connection rather than achievement. The idea of connection and holistic educative strategies supports the use of affective methods in Bevis and Watson's paradigm. In a similar examination of care practices by Montgomery (1992), caring pedagogy is described as connection beyond the ego and is called a "transcending experience" (p. 50). Miller, Haber, and Byrne (1992) also suggest five themes that describe the attributes of care behavior. Care behaviors that are a part of pedagogy and classroom culture include:

1. Holistic understanding
2. Connectedness and shared humanness
3. Presence
4. Anticipating and monitoring needs
5. Going beyond the mechanical

Many of these classroom norms are similar to the underpinnings and constructs of Gestalt psychology, humanistic psychology, and psychodrama with an emphasis on the intersubjective and relational knowing. This is easy to state, but the practical application is still challenging.

Universal Care Paradigm

The most common definitions of care (Gaut, 1992; Koloroutis, 2004; Watson, 1989, 2008) suggest a relational or intersubjective concept. This intersubjective concept is a human-to-human relationship in which two or more persons are affected by their meeting and interaction. In the care paradigm used for this text, care encompasses the ability to be fully present, authentic, comforting, empathetic, supportive, and compassionate, and to communicate a desire for well-being. Today's descriptive use of the term *caring* connotes one who is highly receptive and fully present. It includes a physical, cultural, transcultural presence and an affective and a nonphysical affective dimension. Watson (1989) describes this as a spiritual or metaphysical dimension. An example of such a complex *care* presence is seen in Vignette 4.1.

Vignette 4.1

I am an educator who is involved in my own spiritual self-awareness, and I see an invisible connection to all the students in my classroom. I like to use a preclass ritual for learner–instructor connection prior to entering the classroom and I typically use a candle or meditative prayer as I center myself. I think about releasing all my negative energy prior to entering the classroom and then I create a centering piece for the class. Today I will be reading a great piece by Marianne Williamson:

> Our deepest fear is not that we are inadequate. Our deepest fear is that we are powerful beyond measure. It is our light, not our darkness, that most frightens us. We ask ourselves, Who am I to be brilliant, gorgeous, talented, fabulous? Actually, who are you not to be? You are a child of God. Your playing small does not serve the world. There is nothing enlightened about shrinking so that other people won't feel insecure around you. We are all meant to shine, as children do. We were born to make manifest the glory of God that is within us. It's not just in some of us; it's in everyone. And as we let our own light shine, we unconsciously give other people permission to do the same. As we are liberated from our own fear, our presence automatically liberates others. (Williamson, 1992, pp.190–191)

My goal is to connect beyond the content, and then move into the material for the day using care presence in the classroom that has verbal and nonverbal qualities.

Watson's philosophy and theory of human caring has been progressing for years (Watson, 2008, 1989) as she speaks to one's need to go inward to the self at a spiritual level in order to contribute to healing self, others, and the world. She states:

> Inherent to these ideas is the notion of turning inward and regarding oneself and others with reverence and dignity, as spiritual beings, capable of contributing to their own health and healing as well as the spiritual evolution of self and civilization. (Watson, 1989, p. 224)

Teachers, in order to care at this deeper level, must have knowledge and experience regarding several highly enlightened issues, which are described by Watson (1989) and expanded here:

1. Having knowledge of human behavior and the human rational and irrational responses to actual or potential health problems
2. Having knowledge of individual needs and how a particular person might view the world differently than oneself
3. Having knowledge of one's own limitations and strengths with regard to our ability to care
4. Having knowledge of how to interact at the subjective level, comforting, being present, open, receptive, showing regard, and realizing the possibilities of the metaphysical realm

When nursing faculty have knowledge and experience in these four areas and bring these constructs into the classroom, they become affectively literate teachers. In the next section, I examine how to bring these four areas of knowledge and experience into the classroom through *presence*.

Presence in Caring

The theologian, John Karl (1992), described what it means to be present for a patient, a description that is pertinent as a process of caring for any practitioner. He stated, "When in balance, I am more present everywhere" (p. 5). According to Karl, a person must care for one's own body, mind, spirit, and relationships in order to be in balance. This allows the individual to be present for others. One must be concerned for the overall health of self and acknowledge when one's own health is failing in some area. Karl suggested that a person couldn't be present or fully caring for another when neglecting himself or herself. Balance is at risk from the external environment and the person's inner subjective experiences. One of the greatest challenges is to promote the balance of the individual's spiritual domain, regardless of belief system. Karl suggested creating ritual space as a means of supporting spiritual sharing and balance. So the question is how does one create ritual space in one's classroom? Other questions that are equally critical are, how does one take care of oneself?, and does one have balance in one's life? Vignette 4.2 offers one way in which balance is maintained in order to be present for students week to week.

Vignette 4.2

I have taken time to write a paper, but only after getting my exercise for the day. In fact, I have an exercise plan each week that is sprinkled within my academic role at the university. Weekends bring one day of fun and doing chores, but the morning of the second day is my time to remember my God and His blessings and gifts to me, and to honor the magnificence of His creations and how my mission is in balance with what I have been called to do. Yes, my mission is, "I have been called by God to my sacred Eldership, to lay the paths of teaching, mentoring, and blessing for those around me." I use my mission as my compass to provide direction in my life and to know when I am not in balance.

I take this to the classroom in the form of an opening ritual after doing my own centering practice and preparation. Today I ask the students for "blessings and concerns." These are things we need to consider today as we begin our own learning for the day. I am thinking of having a consistent closing ritual as well, but I am still thinking on what it should be. There is a poem published and distributed since the 1970s by Portia Nelson (http://youtu.be/_enLyy2i3jY). However, here is a slightly different take on the concept, which is so critical for self-reflection.

Growing to Maturity in Five Short Steps

Me in Step One:
I argue with my mother.
She doesn't understand me.
I can't believe she is the way she is.

Me in Step Two:
I argue with my mother.
She still doesn't understand me.
It makes me angry, but I'll change the subject.

Me in Step Three:
I argue with my mother.
A part of me must think I need to be right.
I stop immediately and make a different choice.

Me in Step Four:
My mother tries to provoke an argument.
I think about my choices.
I decide not to go in a direction of being right.

Me in Step Five:
My mother is always who she will be.
I look for the gold in her need to be right.
I thank her for talking to me today.

(Ondrejka, 2013)

Regardless of one's beliefs, it would be valuable to put some ritual and spiritual balance into your daily routines. Bringing this balanced self to the classroom will allow for the opportunity to be present for intersubjective knowing, which gives the students a sense of presence.

Roach (1992) asserted that the key to being present is in the ability to be a listener, as described by Taylor Caldwell's 1960 novel *The Listener.* "Our real need is for someone to listen to us; not as patient, nurse, administrator, physician, housekeeper, or pastoral care worker but 'as a human soul'" (p. 16) (http://www.goodreads.com/book/show/369088.The_Listener is a website full of comments on this historic novel from that era).

According to Roach, listening is increasingly important when individuals see themselves as closed vessels that are not open to self-reflection. It is time to listen more in the classroom, and that includes listening to the silence. Just as silence between two people in a conversation can be meaningful, when you consider teaching to be a conversation between the instructor and the class, silence in the classroom also has meaning. But what does the silence or lack of interaction in the classroom mean? There is a code for interpreting this silence presented by Palmer (2007). He calls it "fear" (p. 45) and it is the role of teachers to reduce this fear on various levels. It may be a subtle fear of not knowing, feeling embarrassed, standing out, or being too interactive with the instructor, but Palmer suggests this is the core barrier behind the silence. Even if this is only partially true, it seems to be a worthy goal of faculty to do everything possible to bring the fear to as low a level as possible.

It is not difficult to see active listening as important in classroom presence—for both the teacher and the student. Presence and listening also have clear connections to patient care. Gilje (1992) examined the concept of presence as a central theme in caring and defined presence as "the ability to psychologically or emotionally be with or attend to a person, place, or object" (p. 61). However, Gilje realized that the theoretical definition of presence in nursing is moving toward "an intersubjective and intrasubjective energy exchange with a person, place, object, thought, feeling, or belief that transforms sensory stimuli, imagination, memory, and intuition into a perceived meaningful experience" (p. 61). This definition of presence is highly descriptive of an evolved care paradigm that continues to escape most instructors. To find this place, teachers need to take risks related to self-awareness and learning in the moment. Imagine saying, "I don't want to be present for anyone, I need to just do my job; it is up to the student to get it." This is a significant reflection of the self. It may be coming from a teacher in pain, in fear, under significant stress, or one with a damaged soul that has not yet healed. In any case, it is a clear reflection of the inner self and the wounds found there. However, there is significant empowerment in saying instead, "I want to be present for my students to ensure learning is truly taking place in my classroom." This self-awareness in the classroom can translate into an impactful teaching and learning dynamic.

Nursing Care Theory

Nurse educators who use a care paradigm are concerned with affective literacy and all aspects of a caring nursing framework. Traditional models of nursing focus on a nurse's ability to *provide care* versus *being caring*. The newer paradigm is characterized by the application of *being* and *presence* and not the application of doing things for someone. The process of being caring is an internal developmental awakening. It opens the affective domains of awareness and is described in many ways by nursing and nonnursing educators (Duffy, 1990; Gaut, 1992; Koerner, 2007; Leininger, 1984; Leininger & Watson, 1990; Mayerhoff, 1970; Nodding, 2005; and Watson, 1979, 1981, 1985, 1988, 1989, 2008). One can see this theoretical idea emerging in the 1970s and growing extensively into practice domains from 1979 to 1992. It has again been captured by leading books and lectures presented by Watson and is called *Caritas Processes* (Watson, 2008). Alternatively, Koerner calls it the *Essence of Nursing* (Koerner, 2007).

Watson's model of care includes the need to learn more about one's ethics, personal self-awareness, intersubjectivity, aesthetics, and spiritual–metaphysical understanding. The Watson model is comprehensive for all the domains of knowing and even moves into a domain not articulated very often—the spiritual–metaphysical domain. Koerner (2007) also presents a highly integrated self-exploration of presence and what it takes to provide this to others. She presents a powerful blend of quantum mechanics to the practices of a nurse to include one's inner sense of who one is and why one is there. Koerner asks nurses to wake up and become conscious to what they are doing and what is around them. "It is important to understand that the science and logic we call reality is a manifestation of the world our mind creates, a reflection of our beliefs and our intentions" (p. 175). She describes the path to integration as having seven stages:

1. Embracing our suffering
2. Transcending our polarities
3. Moving toward authenticity
4. Enhancing capacity
5. Moving toward integration
6. Shifting the focal point
7. Returning to community (pp. 100–113)

These inner developmental understandings set us up to *be* a healing presence—but remember, you will need to consciously choose this role.

The care paradigm, as it is being developed in nursing theory and practice, has significant implications for affective educators who are also engaged in a helping relationship. The most potent interactions are likely to involve attention to knowing across domains—empirical, ethical, aesthetic, personal, and intersubjective. If teaching is understood to be a relationship and students as complete human beings with both cognitive and affective needs, educators must attempt to know them and help them come to know themselves holistically as a part of becoming affectively literate. In doing so, we strive to establish and maintain a classroom culture that fosters interaction, inquiry, and understanding of self and others as suggested by theories on emotional intelligence discussed in Chapter 11.

Harrison's (1995) meta-analysis of nursing using caring revealed that educators believe caring is evident in:

1. Good listening and teaching skills
2. Having the ability to assess
3. Showing interest and providing moral support
4. Putting students first

These characteristics are closely related to affective teaching methods described in discussions of immediacy theory, which is found in communication literature. Hughes (1995) provided an analysis of care curriculum strategies and concluded that listening, communication, and comfort are central themes. She argued that faculty must help students learn to reduce the focus on technological interaction and to direct clinical energy toward the patient as a human being. Educators must teach in the affective and physical domains for caring to be integrated.

More recently, Benner, Sutphen, Leonard, and Day (2010) continue to support the need for faculty development and training as teachers. "The combination of lack of basic teacher preparation in graduate nursing schools and limited faculty development conspires to thwart effective teaching and learning" (pp. 222–223). They suggest teachers need to be able to teach in ways that "foster lifelong learning and clinical inquiry skills in student nurses" (p. 223). These authors do not speak to affective pedagogy specifically, but they are concerned whenever the teaching generates only knowledge without a context or a place to integrate such knowledge in a case study, a narrative, or simulation experience. They want to see knowledge acquisition move to knowledge in action, and affective methods support this outcome.

Educators can examine classroom culture through an analysis of instructional pedagogy, or the general form of presentation by the instructor to convey knowledge to the student. Specific strategies can be categorized based on the five ways of knowing discussed earlier, which include empirical, personal, aesthetic, ethical, and intersubjective ways of knowing. For example, a professor who is trying to create an aesthetic learning experience for the student might increase the likelihood of success if he or she used an instructional method congruent with the desired outcome. One instructional method would be to use groups and teams in developing ways to support each other in a clinical situation by role playing different scenarios. This is a natural outcome in nursing education when we teach a concept in the didactic setting and then have students practice the nursing care in either the laboratory or clinical setting. What is typical, however, is conducting the class in solely a traditional lecturing and explaining format, which is most compatible with a *traditional teaching paradigm* discussed earlier.

CLASSROOM CULTURE SUPPORTED BY TEACHER IMMEDIACY

Closely related to the care pedagogy is the idea of teacher immediacy. The term *immediacy* connotes a direct connection between instructors and students. Immediacy studies have examined the impact of verbal and nonverbal cues in teaching methods that positively connect with students, ultimately providing an affective learning environment.

Communication research provides strong support for the notion that immediacy behaviors enhance learning in both the affective and cognitive domains (Gorham, 1988). Gorham's early work took the discussion of care pedagogy to a new level by differentiating verbal and nonverbal instructor behaviors and their connections to student learning. According to Gorham, studies have documented the following verbal immediacy behaviors:

1. Willingness to praise or acknowledge students' work
2. Willingness to engage in conversation with students outside the classroom before or after class
3. Faculty self-disclosure by using personal examples to make discussion points
4. Encouraging classroom discussions and hearing the students' opinions
5. Following up on student-initiated topics
6. Flexibility regarding the course requirements and time frames
7. Allowing for feelings in discussions
8. Using humor
9. Supporting an active feedback process with an openness to be accessible to the students outside of class

The nonverbal immediacy behaviors include:

1. Nonintrusive touch
2. Vocal expressiveness
3. Smiling at the class
4. Relaxed body postures
5. Engaging in student eye contact
6. Using body movements as gestures

Gorham found that these specific verbal behaviors, when tied to nonverbal immediacy behaviors, provided an effective instructional interaction that had a positive impact on student's perceptions of the teacher and his or her learning.

In keeping with Gorham's study of verbal and nonverbal immediacy behaviors, Frymier (1993) analyzed how immediacy enhanced student motivation for learning. Frymier found teacher immediacy behaviors impacted students' attention level and fostered a sense of relevance, confidence, and satisfaction. Students who began with low motivation exhibited positive motivational changes, but the process had little impact on students who were already highly motivated. Several other investigators found a positive correlation between teacher immediacy and various student responses to courses and their instructors. In other research, Moore (1996) identified a positive correlation between immediacy behaviors and student ratings of instructors, and Robinson (1995) found nonverbal immediacy and verbal receptivity to be positively associated with affective and cognitive learning. Frymier and Schulman (1994) found verbal and nonverbal immediacy were positively associated with student empowerment, which influenced their self-esteem in the classroom, and Chavez (1994) was able to correlate the concept defined as authenticity with immediacy behaviors. The evidence is overwhelming—using these verbal and nonverbal strategies is a way for teachers to connect with students and to be seen as caring and authentic.

Assessing classroom culture for verbal and nonverbal immediacy is a valuable way to evaluate certain classroom phenomena and pedagogy. When combined with care pedagogy, immediacy theory provides teachers a way to evaluate the subjective and then integrate it into other pedagogical concerns. In addition, the overlap includes discussions regarding authenticity, positive support for the student, use of verbal and nonverbal student acceptance, openness to dialogue in and out of the classroom, and a general sense that these methods support a partnering process that provides a *learning-centered* classroom.

PROXEMICS IS YOUR FRIEND

Just as teacher immediacy has educational impacts, the classroom setting itself, however it is established, also influences student learning. Davis (1993) described settings where the learning is taking place as having "social as well as physical characteristics" (p. 46). The type of institution, organizational structure, social climate, and physical arrangement influences classroom culture. "Effective teachers, however, don't accept the given physical environment; they establish the setting they need" (p. 47). Some settings are structured for the instructor's needs, while other settings are established for the student's needs. The setting can take many forms and can support different teacher roles. Davis described the use of proxemics where effective teachers consciously manage the personal and social space within the classroom. These teachers understand how humans—faculty and students alike—are territorial. They create hierarchy and dominance and express other personal issues through seating arrangements and organization of the classroom. Regardless of the teacher's active attempts at setting up the classroom for a specific type of learning, there are no guarantees as to what the student will learn or understand.

> It is important, first, to recognize that there is no one-to-one correspondence between what a teacher provides and what a student sees, hears, and more importantly, understands. The student is an active interpreter of the information being provided. (Davis, 1993, p. 151)

Consider Vignette 4.3, regarding classroom environments. The conversation in this vignette may sound like a discussion from the past. Classrooms can be very *anti-learning* in their structure, and this may need to be addressed.

Vignette 4.3

Joe: "Mary, do you ever have to teach in classroom E? That room is the worst I have ever seen. Two students sit behind a pillar and I can't even tell if they are awake in the class."

Mary: "Joe, I think the auditorium is even worse. It seats 200 students and the last 10 rows are always dark with the first two rows always empty. You might as well be talking to an empty room and have the students somewhere else."

Joe: "Well, I have started podcasting in one class, and we only have 10 students present in the class. However, they are encouraged to interact and create classroom discussions that generate some great interactive discussions."

Mary: "I was even thinking of creating a small circle of 10 to 12 students around a discussion table in classroom E and letting the other students sit anywhere they want in the room, but it is the dynamic discussions around that table that seem to bring the topic to life. I was thinking of rotating all 40 students through the roundtable section on some scheduled basis. What do you think?"

Classroom proxemics has been viewed by many teachers as a given, but others have taken it as a challenge to create new ways of building a learning experience for their students.

As in educational settings, environment also has an impact on patient care. Felgen (2004) and others show concern for the environment where it can affect the healing of patients. Health care experts believe the physical space can contribute to the human experience of healing as well as foster a place of learning. Feng shui has also grown in prominence as a way of balancing the energy of a physical space. Others have called this *supportive design* (Ulrich, 1984) or *positive distractions* (Malkin, 1992) and it has been formally studied and shown to support patients in their healing. Bilchik (2002), wrote *A Better Place to Heal* and she found the following in her research:

> It has been demonstrated that in all settings—not just hospitals—feeling as if we have control over our own environment reduces our stress. When we know we have options, even in the most minimal sense, we feel better. The consequences of this basic human truth are enormously important to the design of health care environments. Patients who can control the temperature and lighting in their rooms, the amount of privacy they have, the number, frequency and length of visitation, the type and volume of music, and

> the timing and content of meals will experience less stress and will likely heal more quickly. (p. 10)

It is easy to transfer such stress-reducing techniques to the classroom by allowing students to sit where they are comfortable and having classes video-streamed so they can get the information at any time and place. What should the students be allowed to control? Can they control the temperature, lighting, breaks, who they partner with during breakout sessions, or how they want to interact with the instructor? Students certainly create their learning space and seem to have a magnet bringing them exactly to a certain chair every class. It looks like assigned seating and may be a stress reducer for students. So when it is changed it may disrupt the equilibrium of the class. A cohort group may benefit by having the same students in its breakout groups so they do not have to continuously restructure who they are within a small-group activity. I have thought many times that I wanted to mix up students even more—get them working with other people—or some other rationalization for mixing the groups for every single breakout. However, my knowledge of small group dynamics would suggest that this puts these small groups into confusion and keeps them in an early formation stage often called the orientation time of a group. As early as 1965, some workshop presenters called this the *forming and storming* first stages of a group, which is never the best problem-solving stage for the group (Tuckman, 1965).

Some classrooms are physically challenging, as they have dead space, no windows, poor lighting, poor airflow, hard chairs, and/or large tables that are not easy to move around. Students are squeezed into such classrooms like sardines, and they always carry their backpacks, which must also be accommodated in the tight space. Now ask yourself, do you think they can sit comfortably in this space for 4 hours, 6 hours, or even 8 hours in a day? Many teachers may have been asked to teach in such a space and are expected to be effective. This is when we need a breakout small group activity every other hour to allow movement, changing the space, or even leaving it entirely with the students returning at a specific time to summarize their learning and present their findings. It is always important to be creative and use different pedagogy to support the learning process when the proxemics has significant limitations.

COMMUNITIES OF PRACTICE

A previous study (Ondrejka, 1998) revealed that even experienced teachers who articulated a willingness to engage in affective pedagogy had a limited awareness of what pedagogy or teaching method they were currently using. This suggests that faculty need to be trained to function more effectively in the world of affective classrooms and pedagogy. More specifically, the results of the study suggested that faculty need to gain more knowledge regarding:

1. Articulating and organizing desired affective outcomes
2. Affective pedagogical strategies such as the use of metaphors and role playing
3. Establishing boundaries for classroom disclosure and student-to-student communication to foster a climate of mutual respect and trust
4. The value of care and immediacy behaviors in establishing a positive classroom climate and how to model care and immediacy behaviors for students
5. The importance of helping students understand the value of affective literacy
6. Proxemics issues
7. How to interweave affective and cognitive pedagogies into a more powerful learning experience for students
8. Theoretical models that help faculty understand how to design more appropriate affective learning environments and students' responses to those environments
9. Understanding why there is value in changing our linear course outlines that only go back to earlier content through testing

The task of teaching teachers is challenging, and we have few effective models that work in our society. Benner, Sutphen, Leonard, and Day (2010) acknowledged that there are many barriers to being successful at this task. Educational institutions have historically been criticized for not being places of learning (Barr, 1998; Boyer, 1990; Palmer, 2007). If this is even partially true for tuition-paying students, it is also true for faculty. Even with the recent introduction of faculty learning centers, there is minimal or no support for affective pedagogical development and related concerns. What we have seen are universities and K–12 institutions building communities of practice (Day, 2004; Kimble, Hildreth, & Bourdon, 2008; Palmer, 2004; Samaras, Freese, Kosnik, & Beck, 2008). The term *communities of practice* was coined by Lave and Wenger in 1991 (1998), which they define as "groups of people who share a concern or a passion for something they do and learn how to do it better as they interact regularly" (http://www.learning-theories.com/communities-of-practice-lave-and-wenger.html).

Additionally, Boyer (1990) stated, "Good teaching means that faculty, as scholars, are also learners" (p. 24). However, Clark (2009) gives educators a challenging warning, "We know very little about how to unlearn dysfunctional automated and unconscious knowledge to clear the way for new covert and overt behavior" (p. 75). Getting teachers to rethink their habitual patterns is no easy task. In one of the *Star Wars* movies, Yoda tells Luke Skywalker he will have to relearn everything he has learned in his past, and it will not be easy (see http://www.youtube.com/watch?v=QtFxrh0gdrA&feature=youtu.be). What will it mean to support faculty-learning centers that influence holistic and affective learning? Palmer (2007) states it will require the creation of a new professional that brings forth the following from our students:

1. We must help our students debunk the myth that institutions possess autonomous, even ultimate power over our lives.

2. We must validate the importance of our students' emotions as well as their intellect.
3. We must teach our students how to "mine" their emotions for knowledge.
4. We must teach them how to cultivate community for the sake of both knowing and doing.
5. We must teach—and model for—our students what it means to be on the journey toward "an undivided life." (p. 205)

To help faculty learn to design and deliver this new way of being in the teaching profession will require new campus guilds—places for faculty learning and enrichment. Palmer (2004, 2007) calls these *circles of trust* that have a significant role in supporting those in attendance to find connection, safety, and soulful personal work. In addition to what is currently available for faculty through communities of practice, there is a need for additional resources supporting teacher self-exploration, how to build trust, and how to support new pedagogical strategies that accept the whole student and peers. Stories of faculty being mentored suggests that in many cases it is only an illusion of support for new faculty, as there is a shortage of mentors on campus (Finke, 2009). It is time to replace poorly understood faculty centers that only focus on cognitive development and technology with circles of trust. Faculty could be invited to participate in a variety of group processes and personal one-to-one support sessions as they make difficult changes—starting with one's self. Such centers would hold retreats, establish libraries, and offer personal teaching coaches to support faculty who want to balance themselves, integrate the divided self, and improve teaching.

There are circles of trust being created around the country and I plan to participate in one in the near future. The current model is to have four weekend dates that are a building process for anyone attending. They encourage each attendee to schedule all four weekends when registering for these circles. I am still unclear if this will provide faculty mentors capable of assisting participants to address their perceived risks and barriers, or if it is something else. Regardless, Parker (2004) calls this "'the work before the work,' . . . Before I turn to my work in the world, I have inner work to do" (p. 104).

The risk would be to attend the first session, thinking that you would appear to be saying that you are not a good teacher or you don't know how to teach. To address this potential perception by faculty, maybe the model would ask all new teachers to attend these centers for 1 year as a process for promotion or tenure? Theoretical models for affective pedagogy and learning would be shared and developed with faculty through this campus model. The expansion of the knowledge would be constructed through classroom research shared at conferences devoted to affective literacy. In these intensive settings, classroom researchers, assessment specialists, coaches, developmental psychologists, and other interested parties would convene to compile, discuss, and refine ideas, practices, and research on affective education everywhere. As I read this, it makes sense that the center would do more than just address affective teaching. It could offer support for a host of teaching issues such as new distance learning methods, international teaching, and much more.

SUMMARY

This chapter brought forward an understanding of the care curriculum paradigm shift; the importance of the nursing care theory and how it relates to classroom teaching; and the idea of teacher immediacy, proxemics, and how communities of practice may benefit a faculty member who wants to begin teaching affectively. These ideas have been tied together in order to build a common language to describe how affective teaching may be played out in the classroom. We benefit greatly from knowing how the physical environment of the classroom and the ways in which we interact with our students can either positively or negatively affect learning. Also, we need to understand best practices in implementing the challenging and potentially risky affective methods outlined in this text, learning from and supporting each other in this educational endeavor. All of these are relevant to current discussions regarding what is essential in nursing practice—in the *art of nursing*.

I am curious and hopeful for all those taking the journey into this form of teaching that challenges many preconceptions surrounding things such as teacher immediacy, classroom environment, and proxemics. It is challenging to realize that there may be more complexity than already discussed in this chapter when it comes to how we create our teaching reality, assumptions, and practices. As stated by Dispensa (2004) in an interview, "The only way to address this [our habitual reality] is for a person to intellectually know that he or she does not have to choose this reality, but he or she can override this reality by creating another reality. To do this takes practice." This is our hope and our journey as effective and affective teachers.

CHAPTER 5

Adjusting Philosophies to Support Affective Teaching in Nursing Education

It has been our duty as educators in nursing to support the learning, measurement, and objective focus of our content for students. This process is required by accrediting agencies and state boards of nursing. In addition, it is what all conference presenters are asked to provide before they present. These requirements have been around for a long time, and we have discussed some of the reasons for their existence. This chapter takes us on a journey that helps us understand what we are doing and looks at where we build our ability to be educators who can also move students toward affective literacy. We already know we have not interpreted our forerunners correctly as they guided us to having course objectives, but now what do we do about it?

> For the true teacher, pedagogy must be something living[,] something new at each moment. We could even say that the best pedagogy is one the teacher continually forgets and that is continually reignited each time the teacher is in the presence of the children and sees in them the living powers of developing human nature. (Rudolf Steiner, 1947/2008, a quote from 1919 at the time he founded Waldorf Schools)

ACADEMIC NURSING COMPETENCIES FOR FACULTY

In 2005, the National League for Nursing (NLN) published *Core Competencies of Nurse Educators,* which presents eight competency domains. They are to:

1. Facilitate learning
2. Facilitate learner development and socialization
3. Use assessment and evaluation strategies

4. Participate in curriculum design and evaluation program outcomes
5. Function as a change agent and leader
6. Pursue continuous quality improvement in the nurse educator role
7. Engage in scholarship
8. Function within the educational environment

The first three competencies address the need for faculty to be competent in affective teaching. The first competency states: "Nurse educators are responsible for creating an environment in classrooms, laboratory, and clinical settings that facilitates student learning and the achievement of desired cognitive, affective, and psychomotor outcomes" (NLN, p. 1).

The specific objectives related to affective teaching in the first three competencies include the following expectations of faculty:

1. Engage in self-reflection and continued learning to improve teaching practices that facilitate learning
2. Model critical and reflective thinking
3. Use personal attributes (e.g., caring, confidence, patience, integrity, and flexibility) that facilitate learning
4. Facilitate learners' self-reflection and personal goal setting
5. Foster the cognitive, psychomotor, and effective development of learners
6. Use a variety of strategies to assess and evaluate learning in the cognitive, psychomotor, and affective domains

In addition, Halstead (2007) edited a collection of evidence for the NLN addressing a host of educational imperatives. With hundreds of references in this text, the reader will once again see a theme of relational teaching, student-centered pedagogy, flexibility, intrapersonal awareness, knowledge of content, positive desire for teaching the content, and a concern for the whole student in and out of the classroom. One referenced author, Lowman (1995), summed it up in two educator dimensions: "(1) creating intellectual excitement, which includes knowing and presenting content and stimulating emotions associated with intellectual activity, and (2) developing interpersonal rapport, both psychological and emotional, that reflects respect for the student" (p. 19). Again, for an educator to be effective, he or she must address how he or she will impact the emotional side of the student as a way to inspire and create long-lasting change. It would appear teachers functioning under these standards would certainly need to balance cognitive, affective, and psychomotor learning every day in a host of ways. However, there is a serious lack of affective teaching or modeling at the present, even with some faculty members in various parts of the country using care pedagogy.

Another nursing credentialing agency is the American Association of Colleges of Nursing (AACN), which focuses on baccalaureate and graduate nursing programs. They produced the *Nursing Faculty Tool Kit for the Implementation of the Baccalaureate Essentials* in 2009. The AACN has produced nine integrative learning strategies called the Essentials to "delineate the outcomes expected of graduates of baccalaureate nursing programs" (p. 2). The AACN states, "the purpose of the document is to provide nursing programs with examples of educational approaches that actively engage the learner and integrate liberal education, nursing science, clinical reasoning, and ethical considerations into both classroom and clinical learning" (p. 3). The AACN does present the Essentials with a host of teaching needs to be met and gives suggestions on how this can be accomplished. "The learning strategies include a variety of methods, such as unfolding case studies, simulation, and reflective practice exercises to assist with implementation of a well-integrated curriculum based on the AACN's *Baccalaureate Essentials*" (p. 3).

The examples provided by the AACN may make the teaching methods different from what you might be doing, but it would not be difficult to conduct these teaching methods using cognitive, affective, or psychomotor strategies. However, in the specific teaching goals listed under the Essentials, one can see some need for affective methods. For example, the Essentials indicate faculty should "Provide opportunities to reflect on one's own actions and values to promote ongoing self-assessment and commitment to excellence in practice" (p. 4, under Essential 1). Twenty-six of the 187 goals or subgoals have affective characteristics based on the literature and taxonomy constructed and presented in detail in Chapter 6 and Appendix 6.1 (Ondrejka, 1998). There were times when the AACN would provide some specific strategies for *best teaching methods*, but they were more general in their recommendations, which may serve the large variety of institutions offering the baccalaureate degree in nursing.

By the absence of the words cognitive, affective, and psychomotor, the impression is given that the authors of the AACN Essentials are avoiding this classification process; one can only speculate on the reasons. Certainly there has been a movement in the past going back to Bloom's Taxonomy and later presented by Krathwohl (Krathwohl, Bloom, & Masia, 1999) where he felt there was no reason to create the distinction between the cognitive and affective domains, as they had a tendency to be intertwined.

Certainly, affective teaching, whether explicitly referred to or not, has a role to play in the education of today's nurses because it addresses a need for critical thinking and self-awareness that is crucial to effective nursing and happens to be an essential of nursing education advocated by nursing accreditors. The most recent comprehensive study on nursing education has recently been published by Benner, Sutphen, Leonard, and Day (2010). In it, the authors make "a call for radical transformation," as outlined in the title of the book. These authors suggest we know three major issues regarding nursing education:

1. U.S. nursing programs are very effective in forming professional identity and ethical comportment.
2. Clinical practice assignments provide powerful learning experiences, especially in those programs where educators integrate clinical and classroom teaching.
3. U.S. nursing programs are not generally effective in teaching nursing science, natural sciences, social sciences, technology, and humanities. (pp. 11–12)

Their findings emphasize the problems being seen in classroom education everywhere that faculty rely heavily on scripted PowerPoint presentations as the primary teaching method. Fortunately, nursing has a significant clinical component and there are many opportunities for teachers to create and recommend clinical reflection into the classroom or vice versa. Experiential learning is emphasized as a key attribute for effective learning using the simulation lab and clinical practice. However, there is a continued concern that our current complex hybrid educational model allows the professional nurse to graduate with the least amount of education of any profession in the United States because nurses can still be licensed as associate degree nurses, and professional nurses do not have a residency requirement before full licensure.

All schools include a capstone clinical requirement typically ranging from 180 to 350 hours, but there is no guarantee that this makes them competent as a novice nurse even after licensure. Benner et al. therefore support *residency programs* as a way to collect this additional knowledge that is a gap between new nurses' educational preparation and the expectations in their first practice position. One study on the practice gap states, "Ninety percent of nursing school leaders believe that new grads are ready to provide safe and effective patient care, but only 10% of hospital nursing executives agree" (Mosby Suites, n.d.). The United Kingdom has suggested there is a similar gap for all nursing graduates in that country as well (Maben, Latter, & Clark, 2005). In spite of all these gap assessments for new graduates, there is no discussion regarding affective illiteracy. The primary remedy by most research suggests the need for a 12-month residency program that deals with communication skills, conflict resolution, teamwork, and attitudes, and continues knowledge–practice integration and knowledge of current quality measures (*RN Journal*, n.d.).

Although there are clear benefits to affective teaching methods (see discussions of teacher immediacy, an understanding of proxemics, etc., in Chapter 4), it is also important to point out that all teaching methods deserve a critical eye as we see continued gaps develop between nursing education and clinical practice needs. Benner et al. (2010) examined many experiential, theatrical, authentic role play, and game-based pedagogies currently being used in classrooms. They present a noteworthy, critical assessment of such pedagogies that challenges a simple acceptance of these teaching methods in nursing education today. For example, in some cases, the experiential learning was lacking and seemed to be disconnected to the more critical thinking needs of the situation. The theatrical and authentic role playing by faculty often brought excellent student evaluations, and thus the faculty member continued to use an experiential learning exercise that was actually lacking in effective teaching.

Classroom games were also critically examined and in many instances, these were played in a way that the students were rewarded for guessing, which raised concern for the researchers. Many strategies that are used in the affective domain of teaching had the potential to reinforce nursing attributes that are not quality learning outcomes for a professional nurse, according to these authors. The researchers found some good use of humor as a faculty member relayed a personal story about her own past practice to make a clinical point. Again, these researchers may be pointing to the fallacy that a teaching technique by itself is a valuable affective teaching tool. It may be that any affective teaching method without the clinical integration or the thoughtful reflection of its deeper meaning, may not be valuable for the desired student outcomes.

Benner et al. (2010) suggest that nursing education take on four strategies that would allow for improved student outcomes. The first is "focus on covering decontextualized knowledge to an emphasis on teaching for a sense of salience, situated cognition, and action in particular clinical situations" (p. 89). Having a sense of salience means to take a piece of knowledge and know how it would be used in a certain situation, which may be difficult for those who see everything as either black or white. An example of this would be a nurse who saw that his or her patient's blood pressure was 142/94; how would the nurse respond differently to this measurement if the patient was a 40-year-old in outpatient treatment, a 65-year-old postoperative inpatient, or a child of age 6 during a wellness examination? This certainly seems to be a challenging expectation for the educator, especially if his or her student's maturational thinking was not at a level that it should be.

The second recommendation by Benner et al. (2010) is to change your teaching, "from a sharp separation of classroom and clinical teaching to an integrative teaching in all settings" (p. 89). This strategy is often lost by having different faculty for both settings with each having their own curriculum design that may not be linked in content or in methodology. This seems like a relatively easy thing to fix, but not when we continue to have such gaps between the didactic and the clinical or laboratory instructors. One way to resolve this might be to have the same faculty doing both, but this could be costly to the institution. A second strategy is to have the didactic course always incorporate critical reasoning scenarios with problem solving and discussion on rationales. The lab and clinical session would also need to have a theoretical application session involved, which would take advantage of time already set aside for clinical postconferences and lab lectures.

The third recommendation by Benner and colleagues (2010) is to move "from an emphasis on critical thinking to an emphasis on clinical reasoning and multiple ways of thinking that include critical thinking" (p. 89). The challenge of this pluralistic view is that it would require the faculty to use higher levels of thought that they may or may not understand based on their own maturational level. Such an instructor might get stuck on what he or she consider to be highly scripted and may even reprimand the student for using *creative thinking* as an alternative for a certain patient issue. I have even heard faculty confront a student and say, "as long as you are in my clinical setting, you will do this procedure this one way without exception." This entire recommendation reinforces our need to raise the maturational thinking level of some faculty in order to implement the recommendation of Benner et al.

The fourth recommendation by Benner et al. (2010) is for faculty to move "from an emphasis on socialization and role taking to an emphasis on formation" (p. 89). This is such a critical element in order to *know I am a nurse* and transition from a student nurse or one who is not accountable to being the one who

Vignette 5.1

I was teaching a course on the professional practice role of a master's-prepared nurse in a course in Vietnam in 2010. Each Vietnamese institution certified trained nurses to practice within their facility, and then the nurse was certified to work. There were certain practices that were universal for all nursing graduates, but they were then hired by various hospitals to practice using the institution's standards—similar to the United States where we practice using the hospital policies and procedures. However, in the United States we continue to say we practice using evidence-based practices, and we also are licensed by our states under a certain practice act.

In Vietnam, prior to nurses getting a master's degree, all nurses are expected to practice under the direction of a physician. There is no patient advocacy, or professional independence in their practice. They are accountable to listen to and abide by the directions of the hospital they work for and the physicians of that facility. However, I still saw a difference between the young nurses who were task driven versus the older and more experienced nurses who knew they were nurses and had a voice related to their positions. I did notice that none of the master's degree students had a "voice of agency" directly to the profession, where they knew what they offered in the context of nursing care, patient care interventions, and how they partnered with physicians for a patient's best outcomes. I asked the nurses in the course to proclaim loudly, with a strong voice, "I know what I offer my patients as a nurse, and my practice does matter!" This was difficult for them, and many would laugh with anxiety as they said it. I am not sure if the same isn't true for most nurses in the United States. Do U.S. nurses really have an inner voice of who they are in their profession—do they have a sense of professional nursing formation?

is accountable. We do emphasize how students are student nurses, have student nursing uniforms, and work with others who are accountable, and thus we tend to emphasize the role of the professional nurse as a more abstract person.

Do you remember the day you believed you were a *nurse*—the person accountable to the state board where you were licensed, and you were responsible for your patient's well-being? You knew you had to own your practice. Vignette 5.1 outlines a relatively recent event regarding the concept of formation of a professional nurse with master's-prepared students in Vietnam.

It appears that the concept of salience and having an internal sense of nursing formation is a challenging issue to teach. That does not mean faculty should stop trying. It means we need a way to teach to such ends. The next section takes that next step, outlining how we may begin to use affective teaching practices to address our challenging issues in nursing education.

AFFECTIVE TEACHING PRACTICES

Educators are using many forms of affective pedagogy, and nursing certainly uses a certain set of methods regularly. The goal of this section is to partner with your teaching practice regardless of why you are reading this book.

- You may be someone who has been looking for others to join you in your affective teaching strategies and build more skills together.
- You may be someone who has been doing many powerful classroom strategies but never knew what to call it; we can assist you with a taxonomy in that effort.
- You may be a critic and have no intention of integrating this material—again, we may be able to convince you.

Regardless of how these methods are used, keep in mind that our teaching methods should be designed to enhance student learning. Here we are cognizant of the findings of Benner et al. (2010), and point to affective methods that engage students and promote student-learning outcomes. The domains for this section are related to aesthetic knowing, ethical knowing, critical reflections, experiential barrier breaking, and some Gestalt methods. In addition, this section offers you the integration of using presence, immediacy, and care theory within the classroom, and what that looks like for the instructor.

Taking the Arts to Heart

The arts are all around us, giving us insight into our inner story. Art is found in film, theater, images, poetry, music, and literature of all types. The key to art is how one's inner self interprets it. In some cases, it is about the statement being made by the author of the art. Although this section could be a book unto itself, our mission here is simply to see how we can use this knowledge in the classroom. We have all studied some aspect of art and literature in our transition to being clinicians, educators, or just being students. Somewhere we were asked to take general education courses in our academic movement through life. Here, we use the arts to explore an expression of our inner selves. When used affectively, the arts are possibly more authentic than what we present to others each day, and yet they may be another mask in our lives that is able to give us a bit more clarity about who we really are.

Literature and Poetry

Carper's (1978) groundbreaking work that was expanded by Jacobs-Kramer and Chinn (1992) describes four classical domains of knowing with one of them described as aesthetic. We are able to learn from reading literature in this domain, but sometimes the inner knowing (affective) doesn't take place immediately—it could take years. This is somewhat painful for the instructor who may have been anticipating an inner awareness taking place before the end of the quarter or semester. Beyond the confusion about when a student might have such an insight is the struggle of how any person might view himself or herself from a piece of literature.

As an example of how we could use literature to discover our inner selves, let's look at a poem by Emily Dickinson:

Tell all the Truth but tell it slant—
Success in Circuit lies
Too bright for our infirm Delight
The Truth's superb surprise
As Lightning to the Children eased
With explanation kind
The Truth must dazzle gradually
Or every man be blind

(Emily Dickinson, in Parker, 2004)

This poem would allow for a host of discussions and affective learning pieces. Some potential discussion points on this topic follow.

- Where am I allowed to be bold in my speech?
- Do I need to be politically wise when speaking as a nurse?
- How would we integrate polite accuracy when dealing with an issue?
- Do I really need to have truth come out gradually? What happens if I don't do that?

These are powerful questions that could be used in a discussion regarding our ability to address peer, student, or even physician performance within our practices. Attempt to answer some of the questions listed above for yourself and imagine having this discussion in a classroom. This could be a very powerful tool for affective learning. There seems to be an endless supply of literature, poems, and phrases to use for such work.

Music

Music can create a forgotten memory that may have emotion attached to it. The music may or may not have words. Play a song from your high school years, whatever those years were, and close your eyes. Feel the old memories of the past come over you. You can change the song and in doing so, change your memory response. It may be a happy, sad, or an angry memory. It could even be a song you listened to during one of your deepest and darkest moments; when listening to it, the song may trigger the same depressive response you had in your past. Auditory stimuli related to hidden memories is a powerful regressive tool if you need to go back in time.

Other forms of music allow your brain to more or less focus on a specific task. Music can enable you to be more open to doing big pieces of work or academic projects. For example, I am using music this very moment to keep my mind focused on my writing. Sometimes the type of music needed makes no sense, but it still works. Everything depends on the individual's response to the music.

Other types of music may not have a memory for you at this moment, but can be used to create a new inner experience. Listen to Kevin Kern's "Through the Arbor" (www.myspace.com/kevinkernmusic), an instrumental piece that may be new to you. See if it takes you to a place inside yourself that may be looking for intimacy and connection. Now listen to Peter Gabriel's "Blood of Eden" and see where this song takes you with its music and words (www.youtube.com/watch?v=wkXeUE5gvRs&feature=youtu.be&noredirect=1). Journal after each piece and see what comes to mind for you.

Journal for a few minutes . . . take your time . . . what comes to mind for you?

Such music can be a powerful tool for allowing students to learn more about relationships, in terms of what is or what you wish it might be. Music could be joyful or sad for each listener. Just become aware of whatever comes up. The next piece recommended for this exercise is from North Korea and can have cultural implications. Some find it strange or even creepy because they have not seen or heard anything like it before. Again, watch and listen and journal what you feel afterward (www.youtube.com/watch?v=gSedE5sU3uc&feature=youtu.be).

Journal for a few minutes . . . take your time . . . what comes to mind for you?

In other cases, a singer's voice can be so unexpectedly powerful, it can bring tears to your eyes. There is a musical video on YouTube from *America's Got Talent*. Again, keep tabs on what you are feeling as you hear it (www.youtube.com/watch?v=pL2s2SWL8QE&feature=youtu.be). Ask yourself, "What is it that is a so emotional about this?" Yes, music is a powerful awareness medium, and it is a favorite aesthetic self-awareness learning tool.

In nursing, we may need to remember what it was like as a child as we start our pediatric rotation. When in a community health course, a piece of music may be used to address cultural sensitivity or cultural practices to include spiritual beliefs.

Film

It is a common practice to go to movies with others to satisfy various interests or even to play out a fantasy role. In many cases we go to the theater just to be entertained. However, you can attend a film to have an inner awakening about yourself. It might come from a romantic movie, a comedy, or a thought-provoking film. In the movie *The Kid*, Bruce Willis runs into himself as he was when he was a 10-year-old boy. His insights into who he was, why he repressed his boyhood, and what he lost in adulthood, continually show up in the movie as this young boy challenges his older self for being what he has become—a hardened, cold, uncaring, shell of a man who made a lot of money (www.imdb.com/title/tt0219854). After watching this video clip, have a discussion about what it means to you. Have you ever had an experience that made you think that part of your adult life was directly related to your childhood? In a mental health class, you might have the students reflect on that small voice they are hearing when it tells them they are not being good enough, or are not standing out from other people, and then see if they can reflect on when that started in their life—as a young person.

In *The Fight Club,* two actors play the same person who is living two different lives. These two opposite personalities cannot possibly be the same man, because they are just too different. A viewer of the movie could superficially just look at how the man lived a split life. One could be very clinical about this movie and see a dissociative disorder. On the other hand, one could see oneself living different lives for different reasons. At work, a person may be assertive and powerful, stepping forward, and very open. At home, that person could become a quiet, withdrawn, and passive personality. How and why that occurs is a challenge, and the inner journey expressed in the movie depicts a way that viewers might relate to that split (http://www.imdb.com/title/tt0137523/?ref_=fn_al_tt_1).

Movies are a strong learning tool and are very effective in the classroom. Movies allow you to teach something that can only be experienced, so why not have someone else experience it and watch that experience unfold and learn from it. In some cases, the flim can stir millions of people as with *The Passion of the Christ* or *The Da Vinci Code* where people put a true or false premise to the film related to their moral beliefs. They may also find a new outlet for their beliefs that appears very scientific as found in *What the Bleep Do We Know* (2003) as it integrates quantum mechanics and spirituality. The remake of the movie *What the Bleep Do We Know—Down the Rabbit Hole* (2004) goes even further, with additional interviews, more science, and deeper questions. What is really unique is the artificial intelligence within the movie that takes you only as deep into quantum thinking as you want to go on a scale of 1 to 9. Once a level is picked, the movie only shows you clips that go to that level of quantum understanding. It might show you something on the double-slit experiment, but passes over entanglement. Imagine if we could do this with all learning media! Arntz, Chasse, and Vicente (2005) wrote a book about the discussions in this movie and about addressing quantum mechanics in our lives.

Visual Art

Visual art can do what film is able to do, but quicker and without the progressive movement and changes of a film. When I look at pictures by M. C. Escher such as his *Metamorphosis I, II,* and *III*, it would be a very interesting question to ask students how they might also see such changes in themselves (Escher, 2000; www.mcescher.com/Biography/biography.htm). Visual art can come from external sources and can help others to see what the image means to them, or they can create their own image to give a deeper meaning to a part of their life. I have seen images of how students viewed their anger and they drew these out on large sheets of paper using crayons. The drawings

Vignette 5.2

Look at this photo and describe what you think is going through the mind of this 4-year-old boy.

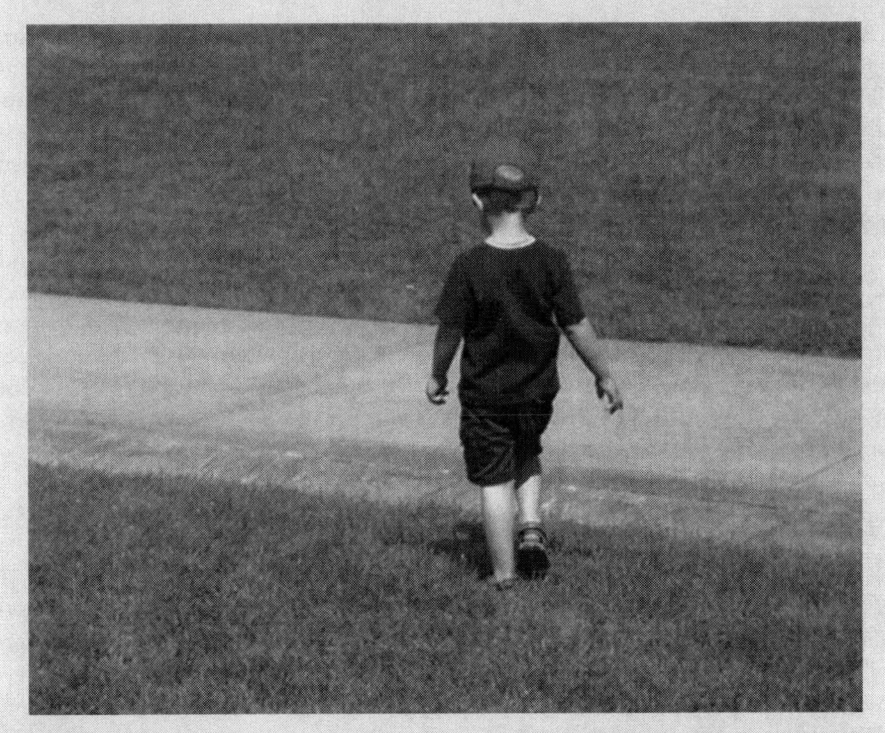

Did you give a feeling to the photo? Maybe sadness? Maybe he is just watching where he is going?

were very telling regarding how the anger built up and exploded, or how it lacked a mechanism to calibrate it. "Photographs are precise records of material reality" (Collier & Collier, 1986, p. 10). Drawings and photos can be communication bridges, pathways into unfamiliar territory, or allow the student to lead the charge into self-exploration. They are considered "the strongest visual statement about an experience" (Hagedorn, 1990, p. 228). Vignette 5.2 allows you to use a photograph in which to move your subjective self.

We put ourselves into the aesthetics when we interpret or attach meaning to a picture. In reality, the meaning is coming from within us. I am constantly creating assumptions about patients based on a brief interaction with them in the hospital. Do we make assumptions about a person based on his or her illness? Consider the image we get from a family at the bedside. What do we interpret about our patients based on brief interactions with them and how could that impact our patient care? What does it say about ourselves as nurses? These tools are very easy to use, and often very eye opening for our awareness of how we make assumptions without investigating thoroughly.

Other Aesthetic Methods

Klimek (1990) suggested teaching care through storytelling and creating an interactive dialogue between the faculty and students regarding their experiences in life or in clinical settings. Hughes (1995) suggested that students keep journals and write with a focus toward the human element of the interaction as a means of developing their personal awareness of caring. This form of reflective journaling offers opportunities for students to know more about themselves and supports affective learning.

Care theorists, researchers, and educators offer a host of aesthetic and intersubjective ways to implement the care strategies that are directly related to affective understanding (Leininger & Watson, 1990). The processes include faculty mentoring, use of aesthetic tools, such as storytelling, visual arts, music, poetry, humor, working with the homeless, interactive dialogue, and use of metaphors. Our aesthetic world appears to be an excellent place for our personal growth as we interact with it.

ETHICS AND MORAL DEVELOPMENT

The original affective teaching work of King (1984) focused on this inner developmental piece. She used discussion groups, case scenarios that have moral dilemmas in them, and simulation games. In one study (Ondrejka, 1998) of classrooms and what faculty were using for affective teaching, very little evidence was found of ethical or moral developmental strategies. We can accomplish much if we study how nurses are maturing morally in their decision making as they progress through school. We have many issues that concern our practices related to abortions, gene mapping for early disease identification, creating life, Kevorkian ethics and life termination, and much more. Case scenarios offer excellent discussion points for ethical considerations, and these considerations will only grow more as health care becomes more complex. Consider the issues of patient care payers, not having insurance by choice, and the resulting care received, mandating insurance for everyone, and much more.

REFLECTIVE PROCESSES

As a teacher, one holds many assumptions about teaching, the students, how the students learn, and what responsibilities we have in the educational–learning process. Brookfield (1995) states that most teachers teach in the same way they were taught and are likely to focus on those methods that reduced their own humiliation and what affirmed them as students. In some cases, the teacher will emulate an inspiring teaching method to which they had once been exposed.

Research (Ondrejka, 1998) has found that effective educators who were using affective teaching methods were not able to articulate any teaching pedagogy or learning theory for their methods even though they believed such teaching had a positive learning effect on their students. Faculty used "experience and reflection" (Davis, 1993) to create an affective learning experience that encompassed aesthetic and intersubjective knowing, and some personal ways of knowing. For example, an instructor might relate a story about his or her first student nurse experience to highlight the instructor's own nervousness and show a new nursing cohort that their trepidation about going into the clinical setting is perfectly natural. Different affective techniques were employed in different settings, but across all three research settings the use of experience and reflection was used more often than any other pedagogy to create an affective learning environment.

TEACHER SELF-REFLECTION

Brookfield (1995) suggests there is a difference between generic forms of reflection versus "critical reflection," in which the latter involves the educator's reflective thinking about his/her assumptions. He argues that "reflection is not, by definition, critical. It is quite possible to teach reflectively while focusing solely on the nuts and bolts of classroom process" (Brookfield, 1995, p. 8). Others (Zeichner & Liston, 1996) would argue that educators couldn't just define their personal teaching preference or style as reflective just because they have periods of thinking about their pedagogical style. Brookfield states reflection needs to be *critical* and it cannot be called critical until we use it for two distinct reasons:

- The first is to understand how considerations of power undergird, frame, and distort educational processes and interactions.
- The second is to question assumptions and practices that seem to make our teaching life easier but actually work against our own best long-term interests. (p. 8)

Brookfield suggests we use four lenses of personal teacher reflection as we evaluate what we are really doing in the classroom. The first is our autobiographies as teachers and learners, which is also supported by Palmer (2007) as a major step to self-reflection. We might write about what led us to become educators and what we originally thought we would be doing. Then I might continue my autobiography about what has happened to me as a teacher and what I am learning about myself related to how I use power in my classes, or how I try to share power. I might then write about my assumptions of students when I started teaching and what I think of them overall today, and what has changed—changed in me to have this difference.

The second lens is to use the eyes of the students. This critical reflection was supported by the data found in the research (Ondrejka, 1998) on classrooms where students were interviewed in affective classrooms and their perspective obtained.

The third lens is to use our colleagues' experiences. In some cases these faculty may observe us in our own classrooms, or have critical discussions about best practices and worst experiences to see what created these outcomes. The challenge with both strategies of utilizing colleague experiences is the need for faculty knowledge of pedagogical strategies from a theoretical perspective as a way to articulate what is happening. After reading this book, I believe many educators will understand the principles behind learning environments and will be able to use the tool created for assessing classroom strategies found in Chapter 6 created just for this purpose (Ondrejka, 1998).

The fourth lens presented by Brookfield is called theoretical literature, which is the thesis of this book for educators. This text will offer the reader a host of theoretical principles that will support any teacher in his or her efforts to go deeper and reflect critically on how it is working for him or her.

It appears Brookfield has articulated four powerful and critical reflections for the teacher to use, which is also integrated in very practical ways into this text. He also suggests additional methods for this work in his book on reflective teaching. However, the real risk for the teacher is to see how this plays out against the questions that must be asked if this is to be called critical reflection. Look at Brookfield's two challenge questions again.

Palmer (2007) has put this challenge before us in a very powerful way by stating, "Everything depends on the lenses through which we view the world. By putting on new lenses, we can see things that would otherwise remain invisible" (p. 26).

In examining Brookfield's first challenge question, imagine our teaching style always being framed using a significant power differential as described by Barr (1998) and as previously discussed in Chapter 2:

- Having one teacher
- Using one classroom
- Not adjusting the classroom setting
- Accepting the 50-minute class lecture period,
- Conducting courses in 15- to 18-week blocks
- Failing to provide opportunities for reflection and other affective pedagogy
- Following curriculum designs that are not always focused on learning

Barr is determined to let readers know that most educational settings are teacher-focused and would not be described as learning environments. Palmer (2007) states, "The foundation of any culture lies in the way it answers the question, 'Where do reality and power reside?' For some it is the gods; for some it is nature; for some it is tradition" (p. 20). If tradition is leading our thoughts and educational structures, it will continue to lead to a profound power differential between student and teacher where intersubjective knowing does not exist. The real test of teacher-centered power comes from those who respond positively to the statement presented by Barr from the 1860s that states, "He [the teacher] is not responsible for the success of his students. He is responsible only for the quality of his instruction. His duty begins and ends with himself" (p. 120). This is a critical self-reflection regardless of how the teacher answers the question. However, if this statement rings true for an educator, that educator needs to realize that it is true because there is a need for a large power differential in that classroom and one should not call this a learning-centered environment—it is a teacher-centered environment.

> Of course our students are cynical about the inner outcomes of education: we teach them that the subjective self is unvalued and even unreal. Their cynicism simply proves that when academic culture dismisses inner truth and honors only the external world, students as well as teachers lose heart. (Palmer, 2007, p. 19)

One way to address any internal struggle regarding these concepts is to take small steps in order to maintain some sense of balance as you enter the classroom. Here are some suggestions for lowering the power differential between the students and the instructor that begins with easy steps and then moves to more challenging methods:

- Bring in more diverse opinions or have a panel of speakers come in to debate the various views so the students get to hear a variety of views.
- Open the course with a syllabus negotiation so the students are invested and clear about what will be expected of them. Be willing to adjust quiz dates, tests, papers, and readings to support the student's best level of learning in that class.
- Team-teach a class and use each other as collegial sounding boards to develop critical reflection in your teaching.
- Ask students after 3 weeks of classes what is working and what is not working for them, and then make as many adjustments as you can to make this a better learning environment.
- Find a faculty mentor and ask for time to present your issues and to get feedback on what the mentor is hearing, but make sure this mentor understands the two critical questions suggested by Brookfield on critical reflection.
- Any time you run into a conflict with a student, check out your foundational concern and see if it is really a stated part of the curriculum or if is it an unspoken curriculum objective. If it is the latter, remember you have not partnered with the students to achieve this, so it is your problem and not theirs.
- If you are having difficulty negotiating an issue or negotiating a make-up, hold the student in the highest regard, and make your decision from this place of *higher ground.* It will give you consistency and reduce the power issues.
- Remember that rules are meant to address what is expected. Not everything happens as one might expect, and that may require a different level of thinking.
- Use immediacy and care pedagogy to really move into the deeper levels of learner-centered environments. Do this only after you have some experience with success in the previous strategies for creating learner-centered classrooms.

- Use a Gestalt method such as, *one step back–two steps back*, but wait to do the *two-steps-back* process until you are doing well with deep inner awareness. (This method will be presented in another chapter.)

It is not an easy process to be critically reflective and Barr (1998) gives us a reality check by stating, "I suppose the lecture is not defended as the ideal educational [learning] form, but I can tell you that it is vigorously defended nonetheless" (p. 20). The question is this: what are you willing to do to change this in your classrooms?

The second challenge question by Brookfield (1995) is "to question assumptions and practices that seem to make our teaching lives easier but actually work against our own best long-term interests" (p. 8). The development of our assumptions and beliefs regarding what is going on is difficult to change even when we are open to change. Your brain can make up what is not there, skip what it does not want to see, or just be highly selective about anything that our brain wants to see as its reality. The more we study what is our reality, the more we will begin to see that our best option in the classroom is to create a shared reality and know that it is still created in that moment.

CONCEPTS OF REALITY

Let's examine some examples of how our brains can deceive us and how we can create our own reality. Joseph Dispenza is the author of *Evolving Your Brain: The Science of Changing Your Mind* and he is noted for his interviews in the movie *What the Bleep Do We Know* and its sequel *What the Bleep Do We Know: Down the Rabbit Hole.* Dispenza (2005) states that our brains are different than computers because our brains can take pieces from different aspects of our memory, our subconscious, or other areas of the brain to allow us to ask the questions that can move and reshape our experience of reality. Our brain has the ability to experiment with various ideas to either answer questions or change our sense of reality. Dispenza describes how the brain decides what is real for an individual this way:

> When we focus on a current issue in our brain, we move it to the frontal lobe and that starts to be our only knowing. We actually lose track of our environment, what is around us, or we cannot even cognitively interpret what else is coming into the brain [like a filter]. So we now have something in our brain that is more real to us than what is being experienced around us. That is where our reality is happening. At that moment, another part of our brain is being activated—the cerebellum. It is an older part of the brain with millions of neuron connections versus the thousands of connections in the frontal cortex. At that moment, it empowers our frontal cortex to accept this complex neuro-interchange between the two brains to become

> our reality. (A paraphrasing of Dr. Dispensa's interview in the movie *What the Bleep Do We Know: Down the Rabbit Hole,* content expert interview section.)

This is easily seen in various types of experiments such as when trying to read the following statement.

> Fi yuo cna raed tihs, yuo hvae a sgtrane mnid too. Can yuo raed tihs? Olny 55 plepoe can. I cdnuolt blveiee taht I cluod aulaclty uesdnatnrd waht I was rdanieg. The phaonmneal pweor fo the hmuan mnid, aoccdrnig to a rscheearch at Cmabrigde Uinervtisy, ti dseno't mtaetr in waht oerdr the ltteres in a wrod are, the olny iproamtnt tigng is taht the frsit and lsat ltteer be in the rghit pclae.
>
> (Referenced in multiple versions with unknown authors; www.positscience.com/brain-resources/brain-teasers/scrambled-text)

It may be surprising that this paragraph can be read with relative ease, but our brains make immediate corrections, and for some people it is actually more difficult to see the errors when they do occur. Some forms of dyslexia actually prevent the reader from seeing his or her own typing errors even after several readings. For those of you who do not have this challenging brain dysfunction, here is what it might feel like to have such a processing problem:

Read the following sentence, but do not try to memorize it or completely understand it. It is not being presented for understanding—just read it.

> *Finished files are the result of years of scientific study combined with the addition of many years of experience.*

Now look at this arrow.

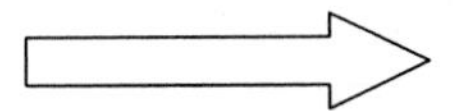

Now go back and read the sentence again.

Now look at the arrow again.

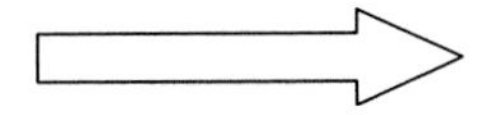

The question is: Go back to the sentence above one more time, and this time count the number of "*f*'s" you see in that phrase. Write the number in this box.

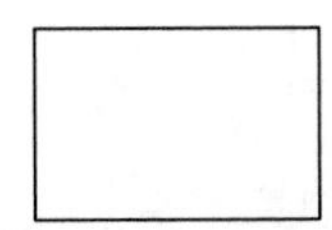

That is it. Were you expecting more? Write it down.

If you ask an entire room of people to do this, you are likely to get a host of answers from 3 to 7 "*f*'s" being counted. Most common is 3 to 5. However, everyone is looking at the same phrase, so why wouldn't everyone get the same answer? It is because many do not see the "of" words in the sentence, or they might only see some "of" words until you tell the person there are really seven *f*'s.

How many did you get? How strong were your filters when you were reading this phrase? I have had people bet me airline tickets to Hawaii that there were only five *f*'s in the phrase because they were that determined their sense of reality was not faulty.

Another paradigm-breaking method used in many workshops to address human assumptions and their sense of reality is to ask people to think outside the box in order to solve problems. One method for challenging paradigm stagnation has been used for decades by asking the participant to draw four straight lines and keep their pencil on the paper at all times. Then ask them to connect all nine stars with these four lines without manipulating the paper, or using any other device. Practice this yourself.

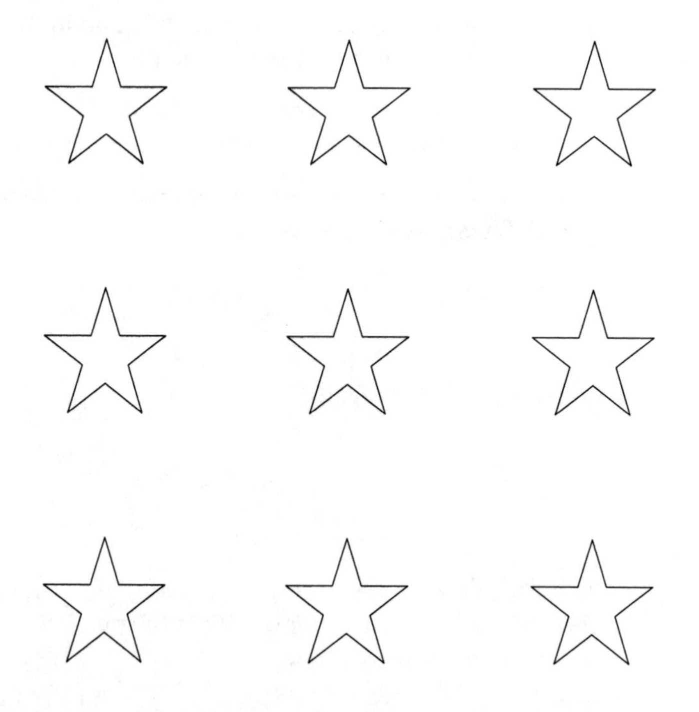

So here is what it looks like to answer this puzzle with four straight lines and connecting all the stars

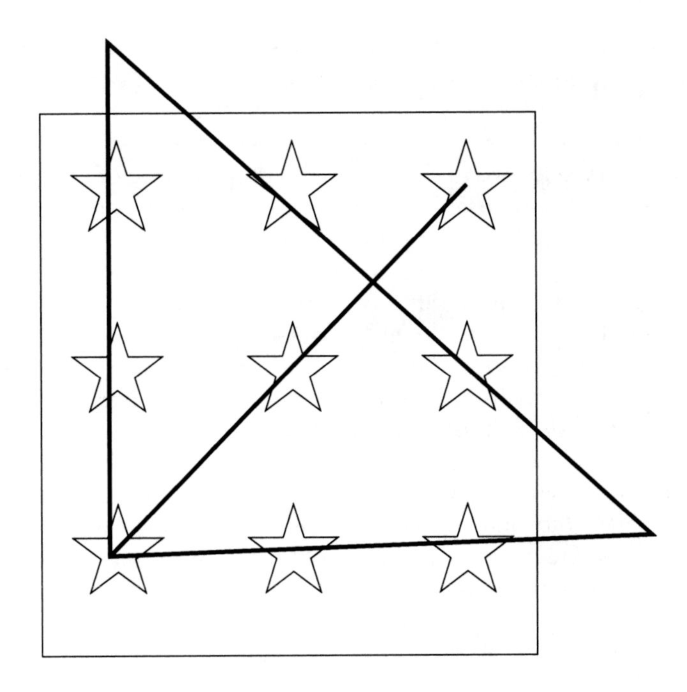

When the stars are placed in a rectangular shape, the brain believes that we need to stay somewhere within the confines of that shape and we cannot get out of the box. Sometimes we need to experience being out of the box before we can imagine those possibilities. If it is true that we are only able to stay tuned in to listening 6 to 7 seconds every minute and we only capture 2,000 bits of information per second when there are literally billions of bits of information passing by our receptors, then we have to question what is our reality and how did we come up with our assumptions of the world (Arntz, Chasse, & Vicente, 2005). This questioning would be supported by most, if not all researchers who were involved in the movie *What the Bleep Do We Know: Down The Rabbit Hole* as well as those who are theorists in quantum mechanics. One of these well-known researchers, Candice Pert, who discovered the opiate receptor in the brain, states:

> Our eyes are moving all the time. They are moving over this whole field of energy—so why do they focus and start to let in one area and not let in another? It's pretty simple: we see what we want to believe. And we turn away from things that are too unfamiliar or unpleasant. (Arntz, Chasse, & Vicente, 2005, p. 54)

It gets worse when trying to determine what is my reality versus what is another person's reality. Dr. Pert continues with another shocking statement, "Our emotions decide what is worth paying attention to. . . . The decision about what becomes a thought rising to consciousness and what remains an undigested thought pattern buried at a deeper lever in the body is mediated by the [emotion] receptors" (Arntz et al., p. 55). Dr. Joe Dispenza, supports Dr. Pert's comments and suggests we can only see what we know, and our brains will be very selective in the process as they dispose of almost all of the 400 billion bits of information every second. Dr. Andrew Newberg, a physician psychiatry researcher at the University of Pennsylvania, states:

> The brain has to screen out a tremendous amount of information that is really extraneous for us. It does that by inhibiting things. It does that by preventing certain responses and certain pieces of neural information from getting ultimately up into our consciousness, and by doing all of that, we ignore the chair that we are sitting in That is, screening out the known. Then there's screening out the unknown. . . . If we see something the brain can't quite identify, we grab onto something similar. . . . If there is nothing clos, or it's something we know to not be real, we discard it with, "I must have been imagining things. (Newberg, in Arntz et al., p. 54)

This leaves us with what we believe is important in the moment, or what we are capable of seeing based on our conditioning. A study by Blakemore and Cooper (1970) discovered that if they deprived kittens of seeing anything and then moved them into light and showed them only objects that were horizontal, the kittens would be unable to see any objects that were vertical. They would walk into chair legs, or anything that was not moved to a horizontal plane. Our minds are very impressionable and it is only if we know it *can* exist—then we can see it. There is a selective attentiveness test that you can take online to help you understand how pervasive this blindness is in our lives (www.youtube.com/watch?v=vJG698U2Mvo&feature=youtu.be).

The subject of selective attentiveness has tremendous implications for the value of affective teaching, in that affective teachers use emotion to anchor our teaching and this is what allows content attached to emotion to move to long-term memory. "Emotions are designed to reinforce chemically something into long-term memory" (Dispenza, in Arntz et al., p. 55). Dispenza suggests that is the purpose of emotion during our learning activities. Therefore, according to brain science, affective pedagogy is critical to any long-term learning for our students.

By now you must be getting the impression that our ability to challenge our own assumptions and reality of the world is an important critical reflection that goes far beyond affective teachers performing their self-assessments. And it is one of the most challenging ideas to understand. The research provided here suggests why it is so difficult to change our old teaching methods.

What is important for this text is to know that all our assumptions and reality are purely useful constructs, created by our own brains for our own purposes. Therefore we must check things out as we build our concern for being in connection and having care classroom built around intersubjective knowing. Our constructs are tied to an old part of ourselves that may have been created when we were small children. Our assumptions come from our experiences that may have been wounding, golden, transcending, or psychologically damaging and are a part of our hidden subconscious. Whitfield (1987) calls this our *child within* and Ford (2010) calls this primitive voice in our head our *shadow story*. It is common for teachers to project these assumptions about reality and our experiences onto our students through our pedagogy and classroom structures, which is a subject we teach in every mental health course when discussing coping mechanisms.

Is there any wonder why Brookfield (1995) states that we must critically reflect on the statement that we need to question assumptions and practices that seem to make our teaching lives easier but actually work against our own best long-term interests? We have come to this point because we are concerned with learning-centered classrooms. This could be our "long-term interest" that is critical to soulful teachers and students who want to learn. These ideas leave us to challenge assumptions and practices that might negatively impact this long-term goal and therefore allow us to check our thoughts and actions against that goal.

Have you sat and thought about your mental reality and assumptions regarding your teaching or beliefs about the students? Have you reflected on 17th-century educators who discounted learning-centered environments when they emphasized the role of the teacher as: "He [the teacher] is not responsible for the success of his students. He is responsible only for the quality of his instruction. His duty begins and ends with himself" (Barr, 1998, p. 120). It is important to know that faculty may be creating the consciousness of classroom cynicism by their approach to students and their role as teachers as presented by Palmer (2007) mentioned earlier, but it is worth reading again here:

> Of course our students are cynical about the inner outcomes of education: we teach them that the subjective self is unvalued and even unreal. Their cynicism simply proves that when academic culture dismisses inner truth and honors only the external world, students as well as teachers lose heart. (p. 19)

Faculty members are living in their own world when they discount the world of the student and what the student is attempting to deal with as they learn what they have enrolled to learn. This chapter has been laying the groundwork for thinking of ways in which faculty can look at their own assumptions and practices that may not serve teachers whose goals are to create learning-centered environments. Possibly the practice-changing statements that were listed earlier and address the power issues of the classroom may also work here. However, listed below are some concepts that may be related to methods of questioning self-assumptions and practices that could support your long-term goal of creating learner-centered classrooms.

- Accept the notion that all of your assumptions are only your beliefs and you should expect that most have been constructed to serve short-term goals of making your life easier.
- Any form of testing is flawed. There is no perfect test of knowledge that has been presented in a course. At best, you will be able to capture the small window of active listening where you find a way to have students hear this critical issue in several ways before you ask them to articulate an answer that is appropriate to the question.
- When a large portion of students fail the same question, let's say 60% or 70%, consider the question or one's ability to answer that question correctly to be flawed because there is a disconnect between learning expectation and student learning.
- It is not possible to please every student, nor is it possible for all the students to meet the teacher at the same place of learning. However, as a teacher, you can stay focused on learning-centered thinking, and that is your compass.
- When you question if a student is in the classroom to learn, challenge your assumption to see if it is real and even check it out. It may be addressing hidden agendas or short-term goals that may not have been articulated, are your personal goals, or some other agenda.
- Critically reflect on one of your teaching assumptions each week. Do this in trusted peer groups where all of you are striving to be soulful teachers, and then let others critique what they believe you are saying. Your thinking may be so tightly bound to your unconscious reality that it may have been constructed for some other reason—but not the role of teaching.
- As you build experience with self-reflection, add reflections using "one step back" and then "two steps back." Do not use these as discussion points. Just let them be stated.

These philosophical changes will impact how we conduct research and create evidence-based teaching as well. The change in our research thinking is addressed in Chapter 6, but it is important to consider how all our traditional thinking may need a realignment.

SUMMARY

This chapter presented information from nursing accrediting agencies as to the value and requirement for having affective methods within the classroom. There is a historical perspective presented that then allows the reader to learn some very import aspects of what is meant by affective pedagogy. Readers asked to look at what we do in traditional teaching and why we continue to do it this way.

As we explored new ways of thinking about our practice, we looked at a host of new affective methods. One of these methods included critical reflection on the part of the instructor, not an easy task as we took a journey through the world of how we create our reality. You were walked through the strange behaviors of our brains and how they are selective and yet capable of reading things that should not have much meaning to anyone. The chapter ends with research suggesting we must have emotion (affective methods) in the classroom in order to stimulate long-term thinking in our students. We started with the cognitive accreditation mandates and ended with an ethical need to provide affective teaching for our students—thanks for looking at the philosophical adjustments that we must consider in nursing education if our goal is better learning for our students.

CHAPTER 6

Measuring Affective Teaching

Understanding research methods that will work on affective pedagogy, affective literacy measurement, or some other level of subjective measurement, requires that we start to think differently about research. It is more than a qualitative issue to the investigator. It may eventually require a completely different inquiry method to accomplish all that we will want to measure or evaluate. We must look at some of the issues that are pushing us to this new level so we can determine if we have appropriate inquiry methods or not.

> Reality resides neither with an objective external world nor with the subjective mind of the person knowing, but within dynamic transactions between the two. (Greene, 1994, p. 536)

A NEW RESEARCH PARADIGM

In Chapter 3 the topic of using research that can address both objective and subjective data was covered. The issue before us is more of a practical concern related to measurement of subjective data found in affective teaching. The current resurgence of quantum mechanics is quite clear in its premise of stating that the observer is never able to separate from that which he or she observes, and this may mean that everything one studies is less objective than one once thought.

Coherent Superpositioning

The idea that what we study may be less objective than what we once thought it was is especially true when we look at the idea of *coherent superpositioning*. Consider this:

> An unobserved quantum entity is said to exist in a *coherent superposition* of all the possible *states* permitted by its *wave function*. But as soon as an observer makes a measurement capable of distinguishing between these states the wave function collapses, and the entity is forced into a single state. (Horgan, 1992, p. 4)

This means that by observing something, we have an impact upon it. I realize that we have already discussed this idea, but let's consider superpositioning from a research perspective. Watch this video again just to bring your thoughts back to this idea once again: www.youtube.com/watch?v=v0v-cvvyc-M&feature=youtu.be.

Greene (1994) states two assumptions regarding the nature of reality that are particularly relevant to this line of thought: "Truth is ultimately a matter of social and historically conditioned agreement" (p. 536) and "reality resides neither with an objective external world nor with the subjective mind of the person knowing, but within dynamic transactions between the two" (p. 536). Quantum theory suggests that reality only exists in relationship. Consider the discussion presented in this video: www.youtube.com/watch?v=LJThU1jDT2o&feature=youtu.be. I have previously suggested in Chapter 3 using *interpretive inquiry* (Denzin & Lincoln, 2000) as a method that can integrate the subjective and objective data that might be collected. This method allows the investigator to use the following constructs:

- Collects multiple data points (triangulation, crossover designs, constructionism)
- Collects any subjective and objective data that are available (blended designs)
- Appropriately assess the data using the right strategy based on the type of data it is (i.e., numbers need statistics, subjective data need themes or clusters)
- Integrates the researcher's perceptions and stakeholder's perceptions
- Brings the data together using crystallization methods (multiple-level integration of the interpretations of the parts) (Richardson, 1994).

We have already discussed the growing swell of contemporary higher education researchers and theorists who believe we are in need of major research changes. However, none of the current models consciously integrate quantum thinking. We are not sure what such research would look like. When it is understood, however, quantum data could also be integrated into educational research.

BUILDING AN AFFECTIVE CLASSROOM ASSESSMENT TOOL

Before any attempt is made to interpret what is being seen in the classroom, we certainly need to know what is being seen in the world of affective pedagogy.

In one study (Ondrejka, 1998), I developed the Affective Classroom Assessment Tool presented in Appendix 6.1. The tool was constructed from the literature by looking at a range of differentiated affective teaching practices. The tool outlines specific teaching methods, instructor behaviors, and provides space for field notes. My research method was to document the existence of any practice, behavior, or action that the instructor used at least once during a 30-minute interval. The practice, behavior, or action would not be counted a second time if it was repeated during the same 30-minute interval. It was counted again if it occurred in the second 30-minute period or other 30-minute blocks throughout the class, but never more than once in any 30-minute block. The goal was to have a spectrum of affective pedagogy being used in the classroom—not to determine what percentage of any pedagogy was being used during any class.

Because this was a constructivist and an interpretive endeavor, I also included space to note unanticipated behaviors or concepts that appeared to be important in the classroom experience. I sat in three different post-baccalaureate courses where I was told by previous students that these instructors were "very effective" teachers, and they made learning enjoyable. I interpreted these comments to mean that the instructors may be using affective pedagogy. However, I didn't really know if this was true. The assessment tool would help me catalog what was really happening in the classes, even if comparison was not a valid use of these data.

Other methodological issues will be discussed later, as this part of the data collection was only one of four data points for my interpretive study. Table 6.1 provides the major taxonomy domains for building a language of affective pedagogy based on my study. It provides what I used in 1998 in my original classroom investigation and offers a few more categories that I would add today based on my study in writing this text.

The sections that follow provide a detailed look at how we can use the affective taxonomy from Table 6.1 in studying affective teaching in the classroom.

Proxemics and Five Instructional Pedagogies

Based on the work of Davis (1993), the first page of the tool included sections to note information regarding classroom proxemics and if the instructor managed the room or became victim to the setup already in place. Did the instructor move classes outside or have breakout sessions and then bring them back to discuss what they were learning? Did the instructor alter the classroom space to encourage greater interaction with or between students?

Davis presents five instructional pedagogies regarding classroom proxemics, and these are useful to examine in terms of affective teaching. Davis's five instructional pedagogies appeared to have four that would support teaching methods aimed at affective literacy. The first instructional method seemed to be totally cognitive.

Lecturing and explaining is an instructional method seen in traditional teaching environments. I can easily imagine it being used exclusively with PowerPoint presentations and being very unidirectional.

Table 6.1

Major Taxonomy Domains of Affective Pedagogy
• Proxemics
• Instructional pedagogies
• Immediacy theory
• Care theory
• Gestalt practices
• Psychodrama
• Empathetic interviews
• Role plays
• Interactive dialogue
Additional Major Taxonomy Domains for Affective Pedagogy (2012)
• Critical reflective strategies
• Simulation and debriefing
• Case studies
• Quantum exercises

Source: Ondrejka (1998).

Training and coaching is a teaching method that is more interactive as the instructor is involved in training activities and then coaching the participants in how to use the knowledge. This teaching method can be used as either cognitive or affective, but it is extensively used in nursing in the psychomotor realm of nursing practice, such as a clinical laboratory course. *Inquiry and discovery* is a teaching method that allows the students to deepen their involvement in the learning process by going into the material and finding out for themselves what really needs to be learned. This creates "ah-ha" moments that are called discovery and can be affective learning experiences identified for oneself. *Experience and reflection* teaching methods set a high expectation that it will be an affective learning experience. We see simulation, case studies, aesthetic methods, role plays, Gestalt methods, and psychodrama all being powerful experiences that typically use reflection for building internal awareness. *Groups and teams* are also a way to utilize affective teaching methods, but they can stay cognitive or just be fun without a sense of inner growth. If there is no debriefing or reflective element to this method, groups and teams may never be an affective pedagogy.

Immediacy and Care Practices

The conceptual foundations of immediacy theory and care theory overlap significantly (Bevis & Watson, 1989; Frymier, 1993, 1994; Gorham, 1988; Watson,

Table 6.2 Immediacy and Care Pedagogy Attributes

Verbal Immediacy	Care Attributes
Personal examples and some self-disclosure	Models words of acceptance and promoting self-worth
Appropriate student praise or acknowledgment	Permission giving
Supporting an active feedback process	Creating a flexible discussion or course requirements
Hearing students' opinions	Follow-up on student-initiated topics
Encouraging classroom discussions	Supporting group approval for warmth and receptivity or discussion
Allowing for emotions and feelings in the discussion	Open to students or engaging them outside of class
Humor	
Nonverbal Immediacy	**Care Attributes**
Relaxed body posture	Uses classroom space away from the formal structure
Uses body movements as gestures	Smiling at the class
Engaging in student eye contact	Nonintrusive touch
Habitualized schemata that is seen as a natural flow	Anticipating and monitoring student needs
Holistic understanding of students beyond the course objectives	Connected to humanness with empathy, feelings, or personal barriers
Vocal expressiveness	Positive personality
Presence and active engagement or connect with feeling	

2008) so I combined these concepts in the Affective Classroom Assessment Tool. I generated lists of verbal and nonverbal behaviors that suggest the use of immediacy and care theory can easily be looked at from both perspectives. Immediacy theory is found in communication research, and care theory has been discussed in nursing, education, and spiritual care practices. The verbal and nonverbal communication styles were separated in the tool in an effort to see what the professor used in one or both areas. Table 6.2 provides a distribution for both domains.

These verbal and nonverbal ways of being in the classroom environment present opportunities for creating a high level of intersubjective learning that has a low power differential between students and instructors. It is easy to see how these practices in the classroom bring about a positive learning experience for the student and are certainly learning-focused methods. However, they may not include a single affective pedagogical strategy. It can be argued that there are many strategies that support better learning but that may not include affective methods. In fact, such learning methods could be purely cognitive using a lecture-explaining instructional approach, and the faculty and students would still have a highly effective learning environment if the classroom instructor was using practices from immediacy and care theory. When these behaviors are tied to affective pedagogy, it may be assumed that this will make the effectiveness even better.

Ways of Knowing

In 1978, Carper started an approach to learning that is as entrenched in nursing as Bloom's Taxonomy is in education. Her work describing the *ways of knowing* were later expanded and deepened by other nurse leaders (Jacobs-Kramer & Chinn, 1992). The four ways of knowing allow for an evaluation of where the learning is originating. The ways of knowing are: *aesthetic, ethical, personal,* and *empirical.* In addition, a fifth way of knowing has been discussed in other circles. It is uniquely different and was previously presented in Chapter 1 of this text. The *intersubjective* way of knowing is a valuable way to gain new insights and self-awareness (Crossley, 1996; Polkinghorne, 1983; Prus, 1996).

The following would be the anticipated subcategories for each of the domains of knowing. *Aesthetic knowing* includes storytelling, use of metaphor, pictures, art, literature, visualizations, music, and creating sacred rituals. *Ethical knowing* includes a discussion regarding beliefs, values, moral judgment, ethical principles and dilemmas, and ethical praxis. *Personal knowing* involves one's personal expression, heuristic problem solving, relationship building, reflectivity for personal awareness, and personal conscious awareness strategies. Empirical knowing is not expected to include affective methods, but the teaching method would include readings and articles, theories and models, and research.

Intersubjective knowing includes strategies that are often subconscious but then come forward when using psychodrama, Gestalt strategies, empathetic interview, role plays, some reflective strategies, and interactive dialogue.

Each of the major categories of affective pedagogy and their subgroups helped to create the Affective Classroom Assessment Tool for use in assessing the classroom. The Tool offers insights into the instructor's toolbox of teaching methods and how much is considered affective or would fall into other teaching characteristics. However, despite its utility as a classroom assessment tool, this device does not answer how effective these processes are. That will require additional research information.

> A new scientific truth does not triumph by convincing its opponents and making them see the light, but rather because its opponents eventually die, and a new generation grows up that is familiar with it. (Max Planck, 1948, the German theoretical physicist who originated quantum theory, found in Gigerenzer, 2007, p. 102)

At this point, it would likely be helpful to examine how the Affective Assessment Tool may be used in classroom research. Vignette 6.1 describes the life of a researcher—going to classrooms and collecting data on the tools used by four teachers in three different courses. Vignettes 6.1 and 6.2 together provide examples of an interpretive study that brought several data points together to create an understanding of what was occurring in these three different *affectively driven* classrooms (Ondrejka, 1998).

Vignette 6.1

I just spent 5 days in three different post-baccalaureate classes, and I evaluated all the various affective pedagogical methods that were being used to teach the students, including traditional teaching methods. After obtaining approval from several Institutional Review Boards (IRB) and obtaining faculty permission to be in the classes, I then needed to introduce myself to the class and tell them what I was doing there. I was amazed at how they accepted my presence over the 15 hours of class. I attended a nursing course, a theology–pastoral care course, and a social work course. The pastoral care course had two instructors who taught separately or teamed up during classes; I treated this as one instructor for classroom affective data collection.

I was looking to see which teaching methods occurred or did not occur in these classes related to affective pedagogy. Students told me these four faculty were exceptional teachers, and maybe I could identify some clues as to what they were doing or not doing to be exceptional teachers. Here is my data sheet for the assessment and what I found. If I use 10 occurrences to set a baseline as my minimum for looking at their affective teaching style, I can start to see themes of practice.

Affective Classroom Assessment Tool Data for Three Professional Settings

Category	Social Work 30-minute time blocks	Theology 30-minute time blocks	Nursing 30-minute time blocks
Instructional Pedagogy			
Lecturing and explaining	14	17	4
Training and coaching	3	3	0
Inquiry and discovery	4	9	9
Experience and reflection	12	9	13
Groups and teams	3	1	0
Verbal Immediacy and Care			
Use of humor	9	9	2
Faculty self-disclosure, personal stories	6	5	3
Model words of acceptance	1	3	10
Appropriate student praise/ acknowledgment	0	8	7

(continued)

Category	Social Work 30-minute time blocks	Theology 30-minute time blocks	Nursing 30-minute time blocks
Permission giving	9	15	17
Supporting active feedback process	17	26	21
Flexible discussion and course requirements	3	16	7
Listen to students' opinions	13	27	7
Follows up on student topics	1	1	0
Encourages classroom discussions	17	25	23
Support group approval and receptivity	1	4	18
Allows for emotions and feelings	0	8	2
Open to students outside of class	0	3	1
Faculty–students outside of class	0	1	4
Nonverbal Immediacy and Care			
Vocal expressiveness	7	21	8
Relaxed body posture	25	24	21
Nonformal use of classroom space	13	29	18
Uses body movements/ gestures	2	9	9
Smiles at the class	13	28	17
Engages in student eye contact	20	24	20
Nonintrusive touch	0	0	7
Positive personality	13	15	21
Anticipates and monitors student needs	0	0	0
Holistic understanding	0	0	15
Connected to humanness	1	8	13
Presence	0	2	9
Habitualized schemata	0	3	9
Aesthetic Knowing			
Storytelling	3	2	1

Category	Social Work 30-minute time blocks	Theology 30-minute time blocks	Nursing 30-minute time blocks
Problem solving in metaphor	7	2	0
Use of pictures, art, literature	7	2	14
Use of visualizations	1	0	3
Use of music	0	9	8
Creating sacred space (ritual)	0	9	0
Ethical Knowing			
Beliefs, values, moral values	5	5	4
Ethical principles	2	3	4
Ethical praxis	3	2	1
Other	1	0	0
Personal Knowing			
Personal expression	1	3	4
Heuristic problem solving	6	5	0
Relationship building	0	4	5
Reflectivity for personal awareness	6	10	13
Personal conscious awareness	2	8	4
Subconscious awareness	0	0	2
Other (metaphysical/spiritual insight)	0	0	2
Empirical Knowing			
Readings and articles	2	16	5
Theories and models	6	25	5
Research	0	3	0
Other	2	0	1
Intersubjective Knowing			
Psychodrama	0	0	0
Gestalt methods	0	0	0
Empathetic interview	2	0	0
Role plays	4	8	0
Interactive dialogue and reflective strategies	4	6	9
Other	1	0	2

(*continued*)

These instructors did not use the same strategies for most categories, but they definitely used certain affective tools in a similar fashion. It seems they were also more familiar with certain methods and these were thus the methods they used with greater regularity. The only practices that were used by all three disciplines were related to verbal and nonverbal Immediacy or care practices. The verbal practices used by all faculty were: supportive active feedback process and encouraging classroom discussion. The nonverbal practices used by all faculty included relaxed body posture, nonformal use of classroom space, smiling at the class, engaging in student eye contact, and positive personality.

My study of classroom affective teaching also collected data from the instructors during class preparation and, after the class was over, related to their understanding of using affective methods. In addition, I collected data from students in all three classes using small groups and one-to-one interviews of those who were willing to meet with me after the group data collection. They all had code names used to track the narratives, and these narratives were later used to create themes. Vignette 6.2 provides the narratives collected from these groups that were later integrated into a crystallized theme analysis to arrive at major themes within these classroom experiences.

Vignette 6.2

Students are a great resource in identifying what makes their learning more effective. They don't know the theory, but they can tell you what worked or didn't work for them to understand affective concepts. Just listen to this group tell a researcher about their classroom experiences. "So, I would like to ask all of you students a question. It is about the class that is just now ending. What were the affective teaching techniques you found most helpful for your learning experience?" (After explaining what "affective" means, the researcher asked for code names, and then recorded the group discussion.)

What were the affective teaching techniques you found most helpful and least helpful for your learning experience? [researcher interjections for clarity]

Source	Data from Social Work Course
Bailee	The drawing and metaphor [of my anger] was very valuable for me. One of the biggest things I realized about my anger has come out of listening to other people talk and say what makes them angry, because it mainly depends on the question [I thought I was being asked] when drawing the metaphor.
Sandy	I agree [with Bailee]. That it was very good for me to see what my anger looked like. I'm not sure if it was the discussion with others or how they viewed my anger [that taught me more about my anger]. [Described examples of new insights into her anger.] I was doing the anger workout

Source	Data from Social Work Course
	book with family members that I live with. I had an "ah ha" that they [my family] have their own issues too. Culturally [in our family] we don't talk about anger. That is the reason why I am this way, because everyone else around me is that way and that is how I was brought up.
Sabrina	I also like the metaphor. I didn't realize how much I don't feel I know how to control it [anger]. It just gets to a certain point and then explodes.
Sylvia	It was the workout book that was really valuable for me. I learned a lot about myself doing those exercises.
Jamie	I did the workout book. I learned more about my anger after doing that because when I did the metaphor, it was at the beginning of class when I really thought I knew myself. I thought I had my anger completely under control, or it was instigated by someone who wasn't willing to talk about things maturely, or someone who was treating me unjustly. I learned my anger can escalate [for other reasons].
Ross	The self-disclosure of the instructor showed his genuine self and was very valuable for me. I began to see that my anger is okay, and it can be controlled to be more of what I want it to be. [Ross described how he had actually been using it consciously and setting the level of calibration he believed to be appropriate in certain situations.]
Monica	I was raised thinking that any anger was destructive because it was uncomfortable for people. So in my metaphor I have two different pictures. I have one of the old [thinking]. [She went on to describe a newer view] but I am still hung up with the idea that anger is destructive, and I know consciously that is probably not where I want to be.
Ross	One of the things I liked that didn't put me at risk so much was when he would role play up there, and he played the role of the client. And it wasn't just me responding back to him; it was all of us responding back to him and that made it safe.
Bailee	I [liked] the way he role played. I thought that was really good. I got a lot from hearing other people. [But] I personally couldn't ask questions. I just didn't feel comfortable asking questions. [When asked if it would have been easier for her to ask questions if the group would have been smaller, she said,] Yes. It was just too large a group for me to speak out.
Monica	I think one of the valuable pieces with this particular teacher and the experience of role playing is that he valued other people's experience and expertise. He didn't have the edge of being the person who has all the knowledge. He tries to include everyone and values each person from where they are coming from. I also thought we had a pretty good small group [discussion].
Monica	What interested me was he interacted with the audience, but he also brought in new aspects that he knew would affect the learning process. [His authentic role plays were very powerful.] He was really good. Scary sometimes. I was going to ask him if he took acting lessons. When he

(*continued*)

Source	Data from Social Work Course
	first [asked us to] start drawing our metaphor, I was resistant to that because trying to force someone to be creative about something personal like that, well for me it was like "ugh!" It was really an exercise of original thought in picture form, but there was benefit after you did it. It was good. I mean, I got input. So I saw the benefit of it as we went through it.
Bunny	I was surprised at the reaction I had when he was playing the role of the teenager. It really affected me. He was kicking desks and walking around and screaming. I could handle that if I wanted to, but I didn't want to have to, so I chose not to. I was surprised at my own reaction to that—he is really authentic at each role that he played.
Sabrina	[The anger metaphor] is the thing that I think about when I look back [at this class], especially with my two big issues that I drew my metaphor to represent. I'll think about the metaphor and I'll be like, "Okay, this is me paddling down the river." I did the workout book. [She had many insights scattered through her transcript on how the insight gained from the workout book helped her understand her anger.] But my own personal realization of my anger, which was huge for me, was through the workbook. [She felt much of the class just came together, but she did not see the teacher as a warm instructor.] I feel very away from him. Like he is the professor, and I'm the student. I think I might have spoken with him one time after class, and he's very withdrawn and almost too serious, very serious. I never felt warmth from him. I felt like coldness. The times I saw something different from him was when he did the role plays. I was taken aback by his actions, whoa.

Source	Data from Theology Course
BJ	I would have liked to see the blessings and concerns reversed with the centering piece. [Classes started with centering and meditation and then into blessings and concern.] I felt like the centering brought me into or prepared me to sit there quietly and pay attention to the subject. I've always liked the role plays because, again, my learning disability makes it so I can pay more attention if there is action going on rather than a person talking. I think my favorite was the video of the baby because it demonstrated very clearly what they were talking about. My learning comes much better just from listening to people bounce stuff around and hearing the professors participate [interactive dialogue].
Peter	I liked the personal part of the class where we opened with devotion of having to present a song and meditation. Items of prayer, or [suggesting something] to pray about, or our celebrations. I like the combination of the lectures and the role plays and discussions in class. The integration back and forth helped me more as opposed to just lectures.
007	It's not just the role of the role play as a technique, but using the role play in very real situations that we have either encountered or will encounter. I thought those were always very powerful parts of Joretta's classes.

Source	Data from Theology Course
007	One of the things I've learned [is] that if you take any classes from Joretta, there is going to be role playing. It is sort of multilayered; for example, you are the person who gets stuck being the pastor, which is always the real "hot seat." One of the very strong pieces I get constantly from Joretta is, "Why is it we are doing what we are doing," and so she is a very reflective teacher. [Joretta's model for questioning includes asking,] "Why has this person come at this particular time, and why have they come to you; what is it you think you're doing [for them]?" She keeps reflecting back to us the same kind of questions she asks herself, and then she models that.
Morgan	In Ed and Joretta's classes I feel invited to learn. I found a little niche that I wanted to explore for myself. I was invited; I felt invited to go on and do as much as I wanted and was capable of doing.
Chaleise	For me it was when we made the clay mandalas. That was really fun and neat. I have to admit, in most of our centering, I've done meditation and all that type of thing, but doing it in a classroom [did not connect for me].

Source	Data from Nursing Course
Jenn	[The entire course] was a good balance for me [compared to] the science-related or skill-related classes. And then seeing how this lends itself as importantly to me in practice. The caring theory piece is one of the reasons why I'm here. When we talked about the nurse artist and things like that, it seemed a very natural fit for me.
Lynn	This class personifies and definitely links together the real purpose of this program and why I am here. So for me to step into this environment was truly an opportunity for me to draw deeply within myself. It is a little flowery for me at times. You can kind of kick back and say, "You know the pressure is off here, and I can start thinking about myself and put my life in perspective, and that is such a real value, and grounding value, in this busy world.
	I was particularly interested in the mandala, which Chaleise had talked about. Also the [class that involved] the dance. [What was] hard was, I couldn't get over whatever hang-up I had that I wasn't supposed to be doing this. The class was nonthreatening; it was neutral. You were never wrong, you were never probably completely right with everybody, but there were no grounds for arguing.
Eleanor	[What I liked best] was all the things that involved movement, and some personal experience that is the dancing was good. The focus and centering pieces that Fran would start with, discussions were good, and they were group-centered and not teacher-centered.

The data for the student groups and the one-to-one interviews and four faculty were evaluated using a theme analysis. Crystallization of all data was used to create an interpretive analysis for this study (Ondrejka, 1998).

Focus Questions

Three initial focus questions guided this study. These questions addressed the three stakeholder perspectives represented in the research data: faculty, students, and researcher. The following paragraphs outline each of the three focus questions and present a very brief response to these questions.

Instructors' Perspectives

What is the thinking of faculty as they prepare for a class in which they will use affective pedagogy, and how do they assess this process at the end of the course? Although the entire faculty readily acknowledged that they included attention to affective issues in their courses, none explicitly included affective outcomes in the intended curriculum. Affective learning was implicit and found in various places within the syllabi. The notion that faculty spend time constructing a pedagogical strategy to create affective outcomes was not apparent. At best, the faculty were able to describe certain processes or techniques they enjoyed using. At the end of the courses, faculty described more specifically what worked and what did not work for them. Most of their comments were specific to their own teaching style, except for their desire to have a balance of cognitive and affective pedagogy in the courses.

The model also helps us understand why faculty value affective pedagogy. It is likely that faculty perceived students' positive reactions to their care and immediacy behaviors, although they did not use those terms, and thus valued this aspect of their affective pedagogy. In this study, the most common behaviors that contributed to positive classroom culture arising from the crystalized data analysis were:

1. Permission giving
2. Supporting an active feedback process
3. Hearing the students' opinions
4. Encouraging classroom discussions
5. Teaching with a relaxed body posture
6. Making use of proxemics and changing formal classroom arrangements
7. Smiling and engaging in eye contact with students
8. Exhibiting a positive personality

Students' Perspectives

What is the classroom culture and what is instructor's pedagogy that supports or detracts from the students' perception of an effective educational experience, and what changes do students recommend to enhance their affective educational experiences? Students valued a wide range of affective pedagogical techniques used by faculty who taught the three courses, but they varied in their perceptions of which strategies they liked best. Some students reported that they tried to take as many courses as possible from specific faculty because they found that person's teaching style personally effective. Students expressed a need for explicit interweaving of affective and cognitive pedagogy, especially as it relates to assigned course readings. Students said role playing, interactive dialogue, and a variety of reflective strategies were valuable for them as learners. Most students identified self-awareness learning tools as being particularly helpful. They also enjoyed beginning class meetings with music, poems, meditation, visualizations, or some other form of centering or creating a calming or even sacred space. These strategies helped them focus on the content of the day's class and leave the rest of the world behind. Some students enjoyed highly aesthetic pieces, while other students did not even want to attend class during such presentations. Real value was experienced in open, supportive classroom climates that allowed them to explore questions of interest to them. However, some students suggested that faculty need to manage classroom discussions more effectively, especially in cases when certain students were flooding or monopolizing class time. Students noticed proxemic considerations when the classroom was physically uncomfortable for them, but they did not mention proxemic factors that were particularly helpful for them.

The student participants were very open with regard to advice they would offer faculty if they were assisting in course refinement, which included the following recommendations:

1. Faculty should be careful to integrate or weave affective and cognitive pedagogy together for the most valued learning environments.
2. Faculty should be careful to see that all materials students are required to purchase are used explicitly in connection with classroom activities.
3. When students are required to make class presentations, faculty should give specific guidance to eliminate pure lecture formats.
4. Students recommended the use of reflective labs, small discussion groups (with appropriate process rules), or reflective time in class to address the affective issues that develop.
5. Students want faculty to articulate and maintain rules and controls regarding classroom process and discussions. This is best accomplished early in a course. The students in this study suggested that faculty manage discussions so a few students do not dominate the discussion. They also were concerned about informal student criticisms that made it unpleasant to risk speaking one's mind. More specifically, they strongly suggested that faculty be very clear with students about self-disclosure boundaries so that classroom *flooding* (a term that means when a student overwhelms a class with too much personal information, like a confessional) could be limited. When self-disclosure becomes too intense, faculty could convert the specific issue into a story metaphor that is not exactly the same as the proclaimed self-disclosure.
6. Students expect faculty to be conscious of, and manage classroom proxemic concerns such as seating, light, and temperature control. Limiting class size might have alleviated overcrowding, the most pressing proxemic problem in the courses observed.

Researcher's Perspectives

What are the classroom cultures for three different groups of post-baccalaureate professional students when they are educated toward the affective

domain of knowing? Although faculty and students alike were unable to articulate exactly what it was they valued in terms of pedagogy or affective theoretical frameworks, both groups valued what happened in the three classrooms I observed. The Affective Classroom Assessment Tool helped me identify more clearly what transpired in the classrooms and what both groups valued. Students presented a subjective understanding of a nonjudgmental classroom climate and positive faculty characteristics. Again, the model and tool developed for this study helped me interpret that finding. My observations indicated that faculty exhibited a range of verbal and nonverbal behaviors related to immediacy and care theory with a few of these behaviors being used in all three classrooms regularly. These immediacy and care practices created an accepting, open climate that fostered trust and risk taking in the classroom. I also identified what faculty used to address aesthetic, empirical, personal, ethical, and intersubjective knowing and now I better understand how these ways of knowing related to affective and cognitive pedagogy. The global themes I was able to identify were:

1. Faculty have a limited awareness of what they actually do related to affective teaching methods.
2. All faculty and many students have perceived risks for teaching in the affective domain and each instructor had a strategy to address the risk.
3. The faculty do not use a theoretically grounded or documented evidenced-based strategy regarding the usefulness of affective pedagogy, but rather use what has been working for them over time.
4. The faculty do not continually refine their teaching in any reflective manner, but do critique their classes at the end to determine what might need changing.
5. The students and faculty recognized the need for better integration of affective and cognitive pedagogies, especially using a weaving method throughout a class.

SUMMARY

When affective teaching methods are measured, it turns out that affective teaching has been a process mostly attached to experience and preference by faculty. If we begin to use interpretive inquiry, we will be able to connect many data points into a coherent understanding of what is occurring for faculty and students. This will need to be a growing area of new educational research, but we do have some information that can provide us with an affective language and tools for faculty to use as educators begin to formalize their incorporation of affective teaching methods into their classrooms. We certainly will need to see more work in this area in the future, once there is some agreement that we believe the data from interpretive studies are valuable and scientific in their own right.

Appendix 6.1 Affective Classroom Assessment Tool

CLASS ______________ DATE _______ HOUR _______ OBSERVER ______________

	30-MINUTE TIME PERIODS					
OBSERVATION	**30**	**60**	**90**	**120**	**150**	**180**
PROXEMICS: Setup and Changes						
INSTRUCTIONAL PEDAGOGY						
Lecturing and explaining						
Training and coaching						
Inquiry and discovery						
Experience and reflection						
Groups and teams						
IMMEDIACY THEORY / CARE THEORY						
Verbal						
Use of humor						
Faculty self-disclosure, personal examples						
Models words of acceptance and promoting self-worth						
Appropriate student praise or acknowledgment						
Permission giving						
Supporting an active feedback process						
Creating a flexible discussion or course requirements						
Hearing students' opinions						
Follow-up on student initiated topics						
Encouraging classroom discussions						
Supporting group approval for warmth and receptivity discussion						
Allowing for emotions and feelings to be part of the discussion						
Open to students outside of class						
Faculty engaging with students outside of class						
Nonverbal						
Vocal expressiveness						
Relaxed body posture						

(*continued*)

Uses classroom space away from formal structure						
Uses body movements as gestures						
Smiling at the class						
Engaging in student eye contact						
Nonintrusive touch						
Positive personality						
Anticipating and monitoring needs						
Holistic understanding (looking at students in total, beyond objectives)						
Connected to humanness (empathy, feelings, personal barriers)						
Presence (active engage to another & connect with feeling)						
Habitualized schemata (natural flow of caring)						
WAYS OF KNOWING						
Aesthetic Knowing Strategies						
Story telling						
Problem solving in metaphor						
Use of pictures, art, literature						
Use of visualizations						
Use of music						
Creating sacred space (ritual)						
Ethical Knowing Strategies						
Beliefs, values, moral values						
Ethical principles						
Ethical praxis						
Personal Knowing Strategies						
Personal expression						
Heuristic problem solving						
Relationship building						
Reflectivity for personal awareness						
Personal conscious awareness strategies						
Subconscious awareness strategies						

Empirical Knowing Strategies						
Readings and articles						
Theories and models						
Research						
Other						
Intersubjective Knowing Strategies						
Psychodrama						
Gestalt methods						
Empathetic interview						
Role playing						
Reflective strategies						
Interactive dialogue						

CHAPTER 7

Using Affective Pedagogy in Distance Learning

with Janice Holvoet

As online teaching increases in usage, it is important that we address how affective teaching methods can play out in distance education. Because online courses started with a reduced focus on personal interactions, Hughes (1995) identified the educator's perspective on caring as going in a different direction from online teaching, which was believed to detract from the ability to show caring in the classroom. If the issues were truly dichotomous, then one might find no common ground between affective teaching and the emphasis on online education. However, there have been a host of different technologies coming to the classroom today. Some systems have multiple viewing locations that are synchronous and allow for interaction that is live and clear. It is possible to employ an intersubjective philosophy that is capable of being distinct, and to bring a way of knowing that can arise in the moment and can also address the affective domain of teaching and learning in distance education.

> Everything that can be invented has been invented. (Charles H. Duell, Commissioner of the U.S. Office of Patents, 1899)

THE PROBLEM

With the growing gap between nursing education and practice, a movement exists to change the look of nursing education (NLN, 2003, 2005, 2012; TIGER, 2007–2010; Washington Center for Nursing, 2009). In order to work effectively in the health care industry, nurses are required to assimilate an extensive amount of knowledge. In practice settings, nurses are integrating technology and practice. Nonetheless, new graduates are unable to bridge the gap between what they learned and what they need to know as a working registered nurse. The problem in the learning sector that may contribute to this practice gap is seemingly compounded by having students registered in one course but assigned in many locations or just online. Creating uniformity and the right level of competency is difficult in situations where the students are dispersed. How will nursing education transition into the 21st century when it is still entrenched in the 1980s where the training is without current technology? How will nursing education transition when we struggle to have the same quality of nursing education in multiple locations? Compounding the problem are the antiquated curriculum models, which are in need of extensive revision; yet, we continue to do more of our teaching at a distance. It is possible that we understand the need for bringing students together through technology, but are losing site of how we need to connect affective learning to these various distance learning models. In addition, there are growing concerns regarding what this means for students who see such learning as less critical to who they are morally and ethically, making it easier to cheat in their learning process.

TECHNOLOGY IN CLASSROOMS

"Technology is us . . ." (Roblyer & Doering, 2010, p. iv) is the current theme for much of nursing education. Presently, computers and advancing technologies shape our teaching and nonteaching environments. In education, Clark suggests (in Roblyer & Doering, 2010) that computers continue to challenge educators' long-standing concerns regarding how we can use technology in the classroom and what might be lost in the process. We continue to hear the rumblings and debates that look at benefits versus the risks of losing pedagogical strategies with technology as an intermediary.

Authorities on using technology in classrooms (Milić & Škorić, 2010; Roblyer, 2006; Roblyer & Doering, 2010) stress that computer technologies are an indispensable part of society and there is value in learning how to accept this as the future of education. Others (Clark & Mayer, 2008; Palloff & Pratt, 2011; Roblyer & Doering, 2010) affirm that computer use in education is purely an instructional tool that has many uses. It is "the raw materials for enhanced educational strategies . . . intended to be part of our path to a better life" (Roblyer & Doering, 2010, p. xv). Regardless of which viewpoint you may take, it is easy to see that both computers and educational technologies are shaping education in many different ways. Computers simply make our word processing less cumbersome and time consuming, compared with using the typewriter. In addition, computers allow us to access the Internet, create great looking presentations, and allow us to program and analyze data quickly for our statistics courses. "Thomas Watson, chairman of IBM, said in 1943, 'I think there is a world market for maybe five computers'" (Kaku, 2011, p. 7). Contrary to Watson's statement, as we now know, our thinking and use of technology appears to be on a logarithmic path and there is no stopping the process.

The Internet created the huge jump in classroom use of computers around 1992 (en.wikipedia.org/wiki/History_of_the_Internet) when they opened up Internet protocol (IP) addresses to commerce. Today, students can track on the web the latest issues regarding the topics being discussed in class. In addition, students can take notes, stream their classroom lectures without being in class, or even send this information to their cell phones or some other technology they enjoy using. In reality, content can be sent anywhere and be viewed at any time without ever going to class. The Internet is a storehouse of information, and global access is being described as "the American consumer's right" (The National Research Council Staff [NRCF], 2000, pp. 3–4).

Ease of information access has spurred new thinking and transformed education at all levels. It can be asynchronous with different students hearing the content at different times, or it can be synchronous where it is possible to have significant interactions from all locations at the same time with the right technology. As we start to think about the many ways of using technology in nursing education, we also can understand how we are starting to decrease real interactions—especially the nonverbal interactions that are a major part of affective pedagogy. It may be possible to address the student's level of affective literacy online, but it is mostly a theoretical idea without active research on the subject.

Most debates in recent years have centered on value differences found in what is teaching and what is the best learning, including the pros and cons of using technology at many levels in the process. These discussions contribute to a rich learning environment with each view stemming from a theoretical foundation, such as constructivism, and intersubjectivism verses objectivism (Roblyer & Doering, 2010; Schunk, 2012). Examples include Kozma (cited in Clark, 1994) who stresses that learners interact with computer technologies to construct knowledge or even have an intersubjective experience with what they found on these devices. The challenge for teachers who utilize computer technologies in the classroom is to find ways to guide that experience by having purposeful clips or *html* sites imbedded in the assignments. Veletsianos (cited in Clark & Choi, 2007) claims that the aesthetics of pedagogical agents are valuable to learning and that these experiences can be found on the computer. The objectivists (Clark, 1994; Clark & Choi, 2007; Clark & Mayer, 2008; Kushnir, 2009; Milić & Škorić, 2010) push back with caution, and suggest that technology is only a support for the learning experience and must be substantiated by evidence and valid research methods before it can be called an effective teaching method.

Although computer use and educational technologies have provided a backdrop for controversy, both are important aspects of society. Roblyer and Doering (2010) list numerous reasons to integrate technology into teaching that include student motivation; instructional enhancement; increased learning; and building "information-age skills" (p. 15). However, how do we impact the students' awareness of self? What motivates them? What emotions are touched by a certain assignment? How are they experiencing presence and care, and can they really build social and emotional literacy in distance learning? It takes a conscious effort to build in affective literacy methods, and even then, the instructor may not ever see the result. We constantly ask for reflections, but in my experience, most reflections are more cognitive expressions of a learning or a belief—not an expression of a new inner awareness.

The more recent use of video clips from YouTube brings about a consideration of deeper questions for the student. In one case, during use of this next clip (www.youtube.com/watch?v=ME2wmFunCjU&feature=youtu.be) as part of the discussion of an online question, students were asked how they would feel working with a patient like this if they covered for the parents for 6 hours, so the parents could have a break. In some cases the students had emotional responses to the cruel and abusive care the child received. But, they were also in shock at how cold and detached this reactive attachment disorder child was. It would have been great to continue a threaded discussion of this case, but unfortunately the question was used as a single reflection. As you watch this, what comes up for you? What would you do to keep yourself, this child, and her brother safe as you cover for the parents?

Use of affective pedagogy in online courses is going to take additional thinking as to how students learn, and what the learning goals are for the students who are using cognitive and affective methods at the same time. The debate will continue and we need to be more creative in our methods.

MULTIMEDIA AND HYPERMEDIA SYSTEMS

Instructional technology may include multimedia and/or hypermedia systems. These systems provide educational opportunities only recently envisioned and are impacting education through the use of a host of learning tools. When a teacher uses several ways to communicate to a group of students, this would be called using multimedia. If the systems are more interactive, cyclic, and even involve e-books, the instructional process is no longer linear and has been termed hypermedia. Hypermedia has set the stage for future trends even though many authors continue to use the word multimedia when they may mean both types (Conrad & Donaldson, 2004; Roblyer & Doering, 2010; Watkins, 2005). Roblyer and Doering (2010) contend that educational environments that are enriched with multimedia systems provide engaging learning experiences for students. Learning is enhanced when educational multimedia "increases learner motivation; offers flexible learning modes; encourages creative and critical thinking skills; and improves writing and process skills" (Roblyer & Doering, 2010, p. 171).

Learning is enhanced when educational multimedia increases learner motivation; offers flexible learning modes; encourages creative and critical thinking skills; and improves writing and process skills. (Roblyer & Doering, 2010, p. 171)

Although hypermedia interactivity is still finding its place in nursing curricula, the use of simulation software is one such multimedia resource having significant influence on nursing education (Kiegaldie & White, 2006; Schiavenato, 2009). Conrad and Donaldson (2004) define simulation as activities that "explore and replicate real-life situations" (p. 93). Multimedia systems afford safe and effective simulated clinical experiences that provide students with patient-care opportunities potentially never encountered in an actual clinical learning environment (Lasater, 2007). Alternatively, in situations where there is no local expert to assist the students in debriefing, hypermedia simulation could be employed, enabling an intensive care nurse in another state to watch what is happening in the simulation room and provide feedback to the students. Such a circular learning process could solve many resource issues in nursing education. The use of video, as described earlier, is another method that could be used as a threaded discussion as the students receive cyclic feedback from each other and the instructor. The challenge would be for students to have enough trust to be very open in this dialogue. Regardless of each teacher's perception and opinion of the training experience, the final test for how multimedia and hypermedia impact education resides with the learner. The learner's perception of the distance learning experience is either positive or negative and will influence the application of future use in actual health care educational environments (Lasater, 2007).

When we consider how multimedia will be used in health care education, many informally discuss a disconnect between education and the practice environment. The concerns include many questions, such as will multimedia/hypermedia bridge this learning gap? This type of education is in its infancy, but the use of multimedia tools such as blogs, Wikis, podcasts, ePortfolios, social networking sites, video, and photo sharing communities have already established their position in general education (Roblyer & Doering, 2010) and nursing education (Billings & Halstead, 2012). Nursing educators emphasize the importance of incorporating educational multimedia in order to engage nursing students in active learning and prepare the graduate for an effective transition to the practice environment (Billings & Halstead, 2009, 2012). How we might use multimedia/hypermedia to address learning gaps in nursing education for an effective transition to professional practice is still being determined. The next section addresses gaming in nursing education as one possible way to bridge this gap. However this may ultimately occur, we would benefit from considering how to incorporate affective teaching methods into multimedia/hypermedia in order to ensure these technologies ultimately enhance personal interactions for increased student learning.

GAMING IN NURSING EDUCATION

Many support the idea that learning should be fun and engaging (Conrad & Donaldson, 2004; Watkins, 2005). Gaming has been a formal learning strategy for more than 75 years and offers several advantages over traditional teaching methods because the gaming methods may touch emotion. Innovative games bridge the gap between theory and practice and provide practice opportunities for real-world experience in a safe and fun environment that is diversely rich with opportunity for immediate feedback (Henry, 1997). Application of pedagogical changes in nursing using gaming will require an understanding of the educator's view of gaming as well as the public's view as they critique the process (Bradshaw, 1998; Henry, 1997; Lean, Moizer, Towler, & Abbey, 2006). The next step is to see how this can be accomplished in distance learning. Not only will the educator need to consider the availability of resources and the preparation time needed for development of quality games (Blakely, Skirton, Cooper, Allum, & Nelmes, 2009; Lean et al., 2006), they will also need to see how it plays out using hypermedia strategies. Some newer technology with high definition (HD) cameras and large HD screens can provide a format for excellent interaction. One challenge is that everyone needs to be heard in the room, both locally and remotely, as students are being challenged by the educational game being used. There appears to be current technology to make this work; the question is, will it be used?

Regardless of these technological advances, students might experience stress and embarrassment when incorrect answers are given or if they view the gaming atmosphere as too competitive. Blakely, Skirton, Cooper, Allum, and Nelmes (2009) are also concerned with creating appropriate evaluation tools in order to assess the competencies of the students or the value of the exercise. It would also be of value to have a staff or faculty person monitor both settings in order to address any process issues.

Blakely et al. (2009) found that gaming strategies build learner confidence and meet varying learning styles beyond simply having fun while learning. They contend that "new attitudes toward experiential learning methods have contributed to the expansion of gaming as a [learning] strategy . . ., [and] the use of games generally enhances student enjoyment and may improve long-term retention of information" (p. 259). Will gaming change the look of nursing education, or are there sufficient gaming strategies already in place? For distance education or online learning environments, can we still have this much learning or enjoyment if students really do not know each other and are in different locations? It certainly could increase competition within the process.

The terms *gaming* and *simulation* in educational settings have been closely linked (Dipietro, Ferdig, Boyer, & Black, 2007; Sauvé, Renaud, Kaufman, & Marquis, 2007). It would be an easy step to look at a simulation experience as a game; the two are indistinguishable in many respects. However, gaming may provide a learning alternative that is lacking in what nursing views as a simulated learning experience. Sauvé, Renaud, Kaufman, and Marquis (2007) stress "the lack of consensus on the terminology used with regards to games and simulations results [has] contradictory findings about learning" (p. 247). Table 7.1 outlines research findings conducted by Sauvé et al. and identifies essential attributes that distinguish games from simulation. Distance educators would need to be able to address using high-quality technology in order to make this palatable for students. This would include fast and nondelayed feeds to both sites, which is no easy feat. It would

Table 7.1 Essential Distinguishing Attributes of Gaming and Simulation

Gaming	Simulation
• Player or players • Conflict • Rules • Predetermined goal of the game • Artificial nature • Pedagogical nature of the game	• A model of reality defined as a system • A dynamic model • A simplified model • A model that has fidelity, accuracy and validity • Directly addresses the learning objectives

Source: Adapted from Sauvé et al. (2007).

be very detrimental to misinterpret who is the first to answer the question because of such delays.

Dipietro, Ferdig, Boyer, and Black's (2007) research identifies multidimensional aspects of gaming. Subsequently, a framework developed specifically for electronic gaming in education that includes five key elements: pedagogy, psychology, media effects, design, and genre, which includes style, form, and game content. Faculty wanting to integrate gaming in distance learning will want to address each of the five elements and include an assessment of the gaming's software/hardware capabilities.

Even though games can be viewed as a viable teaching strategy, literature provides conflicting views. Blakely et al. (2009) provide a list of potential positive outcomes from the use of games in nursing education (see Table 7.2). Royse and Newton (2007) contend that gaming is an innovative teaching strategy and improves nursing student learning outcomes, whereas Benner, Sutphen, Leonard, and Day (2010) state:

> Although the students' attention is gained through games, the quality of their attentiveness may fall short of serious engagement with the practice of nursing. Whether the teacher intends it or not, games can reinforce the idea that guessing is acceptable and that memorization is the major learning goal in nursing education. (p. 74)

It would seem necessary for faculty to be concerned with what the exercise means to the student and their own self-awareness and learning. If there were guided reflection steps to look at what just occurred and what may be hidden to the student during the exercise, then the reflection might allow for a deeper sense of what was previously hidden to the student. We may rethink the value of putting gaming strategies into distance learning when it adds the component of heavy competition as well. Benner et al. (2010) warn educators there may be unintended consequences when we turn education into competition behaviors. For example, consider how competition could have negative impacts on learning. Yet, others list possible benefits.

Table 7.2 Advantages of Gaming

• Reduces stress and anxiety
• Stimulates interaction
• Reduces monotonous lessons
• Promotes teamwork
• Creates a conductive environment for increased learning and retention of knowledge
• Enhances motivation
• Promotes a relaxed learning environment
• Adds entertainment

Source: Adapted from Henderson as cited in Blakely et al. (2009, p. 261).

Pardue, Tagliareni, and Valiga (2005) list several recommendations supporting innovation in nursing (including gaming) that include:

- Explore new pedagogies to enhance nursing education, including gaming
- Review current research supporting (or not supporting) gaming, to provide evidence and inform decisions regarding new pedagogies that bridge education and practice gaps
- Engage in dialogue with peers, students, and nursing practice colleagues to design, incorporate, and evaluate gaming strategies that enhance student learning outcomes, meet students' needs, and prepare graduates for today's health care environment
- Conduct pedagogical research to document the effectiveness and meaningfulness of gaming innovations that are occurring in nursing education (p. 2).

Table 7.3 outlines seven characteristics of nurses positively influenced by gaming.

It is clear that gaming in nursing education has strong support for and against its use and yet the issue may be a lack of method that allows for effective learning, affective literacy, and positive personal growth to occur. This subject does need additional research and reflection on the part of the instructors using it.

CHEATING WITH TECHNOLOGY

Another important consideration regarding the use of distance education is the idea of cheating. Technology is contributing to a student's ability to bypass the learning process completely. One site (http://www.writework.com)

Table 7.3 Characteristics of Nurses Influenced by Gaming

1. Heterogeneous population—Gaming allows the interaction of nurses from different backgrounds to learn from each other's experience.
2. Active learning—Games promote an active learning style and offer immediate feedback.
3. Compassion—Nurses need empathy skills to provide support and understanding. Games provide a relaxed environment to develop these abilities.
4. Complex work environment—Provides opportunities for nurses to understand the intricacies of their work in a controlled atmosphere.
5. Time—Increases the amount of experiences available compared to other learning formats.
6. Motivation—Promotes motivational learning through interaction, individual learning, and immediate feedback.
7. Communication—Enhanced through gaming interaction and group discussion.

Source: Adapted from Fuszard as cited in Blakely et al. (2009, p. 260).

has over 115,000 essays, research papers, and book reports that students can plagiarize. This certainly goes far beyond a concern regarding the student having an experiential or affective learning experience. Our worst-case scenario is the use of technology to avoid all learning or eliminate any form of examination measurement as an effective tool for assessing our students. There are hosts of strategies that can be employed to cheat in school, and technology is a major player in such behavior. Recent articles describe cheating as:

> Academic cheating is prevalent worldwide and has in fact seen a steady increase in recent decades as the digital era facilitates more sophisticated and creative cheating methods. (Kahn, in Moussly, 2012)

- Buying a paper from an Internet site
- Obtaining a copy of the test banks
- Sharing homework answers via IMs, e-mail, text messaging, or invisible ear pieces
- Using a whiteboard to share answers
- Having another student write a paper
- Cutting and pasting text from the Internet without citing it
- Using sample essays from the Internet
- Programming notes or storing definitions into a calculator
- Taking and/or sending a cell phone picture of test material or notes
- Video recording lectures with cell phones and replaying during test
- Surfing the web for answers during a test

- Using a pager to receive information during a test
- Viewing notes on your electronic device during a test
- Accessing the teacher's computer files
- Using a watch, eraser, or pen to hold notes
- Using a laser pen to "write" and send answers (Fleming, n.d.; Yaccino, 2008)

Khan (in Moussly, 2012) found that more than 78% of the students surveyed at the University of Wollongong in Dubai "admitted to engaging in some form of cheating. . . . It raises serious concern regarding the academic integrity of the graduates being churned out to the UAE's workforce" (Moussly, 2012, para. 3). Khan states, "Academic cheating is prevalent worldwide and has in fact seen a steady increase in recent decades as the digital era facilitates more sophisticated and creative cheating methods" (Moussly, 2012, para. 1).

In another example, Harvard University has recently begun investigating 250 students for cheating on a final take-home examination. "'These allegations, if proven, represent totally unacceptable behavior that betrays the trust upon which intellectual inquiry at Harvard depends," said Harvard University President Drew Faust (IANS, 2012, para. 5). A YouTube (2010, November 23) video clip shows just how serious issues can become in a single University of Central Florida class where the entire test bank was compromised (www.youtube.com/watch?v=7AdYAUe8q9w&feature=youtu.be).

Cheating may be a more subtle symptom of what we might call a low-risk game, or something of minimal importance when our values do not kick in as they would if cheating was found on a really important exam or paper. Neal Conan, host of NPR radio's *Talk of the Nation*, conducted a live broadcast on what people believe about cheating. Conan's guest was Dan Ariely who has conducted research on what drives people to cheat (Conan, September 24, 2012). Based on the calls and the research by Ariely (2012), it is obvious that there is a serious issue with what callers considered to be small issues versus big issues related to cheating. Ariely states:

> And what we find is that lots of people cheat a little bit. . . . [I]t's true that there are few big cheaters out there and it's really terrible, but the capacity to cheat a little bit and feel good about ourselves is really much more common than we think it is. And because of that, it's much more dangerous. And because of that, we need to think about how we engineered the environment [we live in]—especially around politics and the business world—not to let that cheating kind of blossom and create tremendous devastation. . . . And I think we all do this partitioning to some degree [i.e., partition of life into things that are outside and inside the realm of importance], that there are some areas of life that we can behave immorally, but we somehow don't see the carryover to other areas of life. We just kind of partition it

> and set it aside as something that is just acceptable in its own domain. (pp. 4–5)

It is apparent that morally driven and value-based students will see cheating as a *big* issue when it affects family, financial losses, and a breakdown of some important system. However, in the smaller realm (e.g., online games, music downloading, cheating at cards) where cheating does not seem to cause real harm, it is seen as *small* cheating and is not really a moral issue for them. It is seen as being not very important. This can easily be transported to student thinking in schools, where it doesn't really hurt anyone and cheating will make their life improve—that is, it will take less time and can improve their grades.

Roblyer and Doering (2010) identify plagiarism as a major pitfall in the use of technology as students use the Internet to complement knowledge acquisition. Neville's (2007) research provides evidence that 20% to 25% of students admittedly plagiarize. In a student survey of student perceptions, Neville (2007) states, "[Seventy] percent of fellow classmates copy content from books and the Internet without citing the source" (p. 29).

Future technologies will most likely bring additional educational concerns to the forefront. Kaku (2011), a futurist, discusses current and future technology that is going to be a major threat to how teachers will be able to control cheating. He believes that the computer will even disappear from our language because we will be accessing data chips in everything we do; the computer will not be needed to coordinate information into useful data. He describes virtual retinal display (VRD), which can send an image directly to the retina with something like eyeglasses, as seen in *Mission Impossible* movies. Such acuity can see the full screen of a computer with clarity. The University of Washington has been working on this technology since 1991; they can already create crystal clear images with a pixel resolution of 1600 × 1200. Kaku also provides current research on Internet contact lenses, where the contact lenses will be able to do the same thing as the eyeglasses. We could also have thought-activation digital chips that would allow a student to think about an answer to a question needed on an exam and it would show up on his or her contact lens. Imagine a learning assignment that needs completion in the classroom; I could think about the paper as well as the Web, and immediately receive a copy on a processing chip in my glasses or pocket that sends it to my contact lens. I could even write this paper while you are watching me as it would be visible to only me.

Kaku (2011) does not discuss the abuse of such technology, but it is not difficult to see the future when educators will need to deal with 2030 technology, and use technology detectors before a student can enter the test-taking room. Futuristic portrayals may include centers that have *disturbance fields* around them to prevent

> Of course, science is a double-edged sword: it creates as many problems as it solves, but always on a higher level. (Kaku, 2011, p. 16)

external knowledge sources from entering the room in any form, or from functioning once the student enters the room. Is it comprehensible that such centers might be leased by universities around the country for student in-seat testing, as there may be no other method for measuring student knowledge on a given subject.

SUMMARY

Technology will continue to drive the future of nursing education, whether education occurs in one location, multiple locations, or in every student's home. However, strong emphasis is placed on the need for additional research that informs the use of technologies in education—especially gaming and cheating. The review of literature is controversial regarding the use of gaming (and other forms of technology) pedagogy. Additionally, controls on cheating will continue to be a challenge as technology enhances the future of education. For distance/online learning, the demands on faculty will continue to soar. In order to surmount these challenges, nursing educators must collaborate with professional practice partners to ensure that these technologies are capable of satisfying the new-graduate *RN-to-practice knowledge gap*. Together, we must envision and shape the future, as distance learning becomes an absolute in both practice and education settings. If we unite and work proactively, we can meet this challenge.

CHAPTER 8

Moving From Presentation Slides to Affective Teaching at Conferences

POWERPOINT EXPERIENCES

I was attending a national conference in 2004, and on the third day, I realized every presentation used the following elements:

1. Measurable objectives
2. PowerPoint presentations
3. Lecture-listen-stop format with questions at the end in some cases

> Teachers in classrooms often rely heavily on automated presentation software and use pedagogical strategies that are significantly less effective than teachers generally use in clinical settings and skills labs where knowledge acquisition use are more integrated. (Benner, Sutphen, Leonard, & Day, 2010, p. 65)

Does this sound familiar? In 2011, I attended and presented at another national conference. Faculty were given the following format and told to stick to it:

1. Have one or two measurable objectives
2. Present for 20 to 25 minutes
3. Allow time for questions
4. Use a PowerPoint presentation
5. Provide handouts for the attendees
6. Start and end with a slide of your objectives

I was compliant, and amazed how difficult it was. I intended to include a lecture–discussion method during my 20- to 25-minute talk, knowing that the audience would be limited to approximately 75 attendees. Many attendees came in late because this conference used a rapid-fire method of introducing three presenters every 75 minutes with a 15-minute break between sessions. If you were the first presenter, only two thirds of the audience heard your presentation. It takes time to engage attendees who come in late, and to move from the content of your presentation, to engaging the audience with participation strategies. I learned that I do not enjoy attending or presenting at a conference if my presentation has to be fully content driven. I do not believe that one can engage the audience in tight presentation time frames, and there are some habitual behaviors of students and conference attendees that are challenging for my style of teaching. Many come in late, seem lost, and then distract others. Although this type of behavior can be reduced in the classroom through attendance policies, it is rampant at conference presentations.

With an opportunity to present at a different conference later in 2011, I was fearful of losing my audience because I was going to integrate hospital metric data, patient satisfaction goals, and how we use data inappropriately to mislead our audiences. The good part regarding this presentation was that I had 90 minutes and I was asked to submit a PowerPoint for a booklet going to the attendees during the conference—which I did. You may be wondering if I enjoyed giving this 90-minute presentation. I did enjoy it, as I stretched the audience to interact in ways that shook their belief system and challenged their habitual thinking. It was the most affective presentation I have ever attempted, and the audience left grappling with the fact that what has always been assumed as reality in patient satisfaction methods is actually more of an illusion.

In the past, presenter's presentations were handcuffed by PowerPoint, but it no longer needs to be this way. The issue is really about the presenter's desire to connect, to stretch the audience, or to quickly create some interactive learning in the midst of the presentation. Such problems are not seen just in conferences, but in the classroom as well. It may be tied to our need for being objective, clear, directional, and goal oriented, which may have started with our view of creating measurable objectives for all our courses and presentations. Tylerian objectivism (Tyler, 1949) was a foundational pre-empting for nurses creating presentation objectives. We were taught to use a measurable verb—will know, describe, provide, compare, will use, and so forth. However, I believe we have incorrectly interpreted Tyler's push for objectives in teaching. His writings do not support pure objectivism for purposes of measurement, as mentioned in Chapter 2. To reiterate, Tyler was attempting to integrate the subjective elements into the objective and states:

> Education is a process of changing the behavior patterns of people. This is using behavior in the broad sense to include thinking and feeling as well as overt action. When education is viewed in this way it is clear that educational objectives then represent the kinds

of change in behavior that an educational institution seeks to bring about in its students. (pp. 5–6)

His examples mix subjective and objective learning together, and yet we have sterilized this to the point of killing the subjective element. It appears that we really do fear the subjective as suggested by Palmer (2007), which leaves us with holes in our presentations.

It would be interesting to study professional conference presentations the way we have studied the classroom. We would likely see a serious problem with how the presentations are perceived by the audience, which would support my bias that we would benefit from having affective or other creative methods used during conference presentations. One recent change is the use of musicians performing between the speakers and getting the audience involved or allowing them to mindfully go to peaceful places as they listen to the music.

FOUR STAGES OF POWERPOINT USAGE

Paradi's (2010) *102 Tips to Communicate More Effectively Using PowerPoint* demonstrates how to make a more powerful impact with a presentation by using tailored structure, design, content, and delivery. In addition, he suggests websites to improve your use of PowerPoint (www.thinkoutsidetheslide.com and pptideas.blogspot.com/2012/07/presentation-tip-how-to-use-about-us.html).

While watching his video, I noticed that his use of PowerPoint made his presentations better, but he did not move toward an affective teaching experience. However, I did learn why so many PowerPoint presentations are not good teaching tools.

Paradi makes a distinction in how we see presenters use their PowerPoint. These are his four stages. The first is a script-reading lecture, where the person presents everything he or she wants to say on the slides. It is pure reading and sometimes the presenter often does this with his or her back turned to the audience. This form of presentation lacks connection, is not well received, and yet is seen regularly at conferences, although it is becoming less frequent (see Figure 8.1).

The second stage resembles speaker's notes and is really for the presenter, not the audience. This topical outline tells the speaker he or she is covering the right material and in the correct order. It is all text and is equivalent to *instructor-centered* teaching. I have used this method many times because it is easy to use and allows me to add content, which allows the speaker to "flesh out" the outline (see Figure 8.2).

The third stage is called visual noise with so much going on that the audience is not really able to grasp what the slide is presenting. In addition, there may be added sound effects to the animations in the slide or some other feature that is distracting to the content. For example, see Figure 8.3.

All Professions Have Accountabilities

PATIENTS AND FAMILIES ARE THE
REASON WE EXIST

Caring is critical in helping people maintain health, promote healing, adapt to stressful experiences, and in supporting a dignified death. We believvw self-determination is a fundamental human right. Our understanding of caring is based on Jean Watson's Human Caring Theory.

This means that:

- A nurse/patient relationship is established based on personal presence and rapport.
- Caring involves acts and attitudes of critical thinking, clinical competency, compassion, respect, listening, and acceptance.
- Caring is maintained and kept in balance with technology in an envoronment where change occures at an accelerated place.
- Patients are valued as individuals and partners who possess unique knowledge and information and are active participants in their health care decisions.
- Patients' rights to privacy and confidentiality are respected and maintained.
- Individual support systems important to the patient are recognized, valued, and supported.

Figure 8.1 Full-script slide.

Nursing's Two Domains: Client and Profession Focused

Nursing Process

- Assesment
- Diagnosis
- Outcomes identified
- Implementation
- Evaluation

Professional Expectation

- Quality of practice model
- Life-long learning
- Professional practice evaluation process
- Function collegially and collaboratively
- Use an ethical practice
- Use research and EBP
- Resource utilization
- Leadership

Figure 8.2 Outline slide.

Sometimes it takes its toll and we lose our balance
FRED = Frantically Running Everywhere Daily
more patients
Communication
FRED
No Time
Clinical
Knowledge

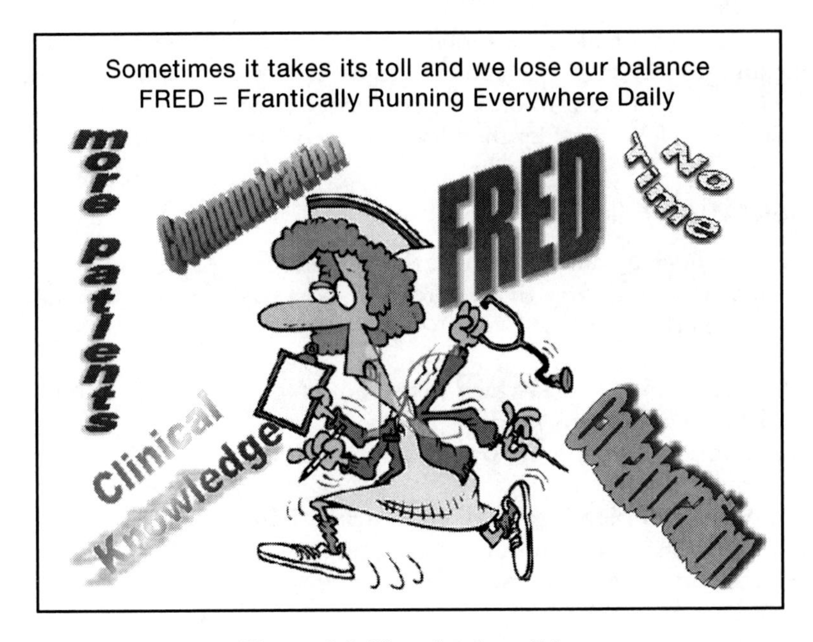

Figure 8.3 Visual noise slide.

The fourth stage is used and advocated by Paradi, who believes this is the best type of presentation method. It is considered a persuasion-visual method. It provides something to remember and then offers a visual aid to make it memorable. Figure 8.4 is an example of such a slide.

You Have to be willing to learn new things

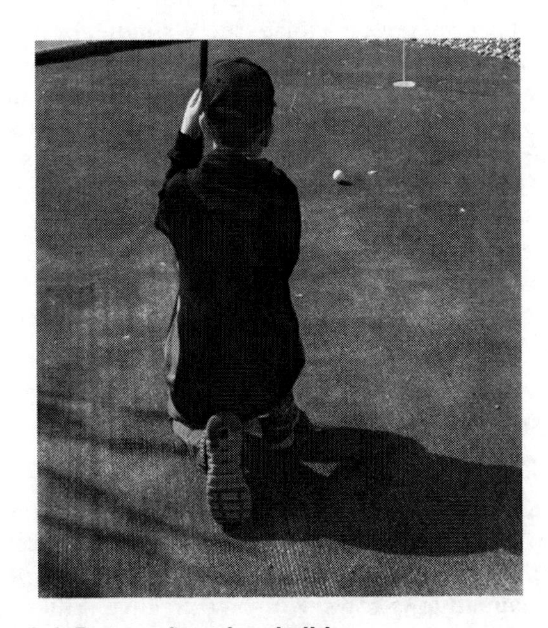

Figure 8.4 Persuasion-visual slide.

Although Figure 8.4 makes the audience think about what the presenter is discussing and thus engages the audience more effectively, it still does not offer an affective presentation. In order to go deeper to achieve affective presentations, I'd like to first consider the idea of presentation etiquette.

PRESENTATION ETIQUETTE

Many presenters may not be aware of the guidelines of presentation etiquette, so it is beneficial to outline those here. The most basic presentation etiquette may be summed up as:

- Remember the 6 × 7 rule, which states: no more than 6 lines or bullets per slide, and no more than 7 words per line.
- Use caution with flamboyant backgrounds and strange lettering (e.g., Comic Sans typeface).
- Avoid poor color blends from type to background.
- Don't use animation or transitions with text.
- Use a real video clip to show a complex issue.
- NEVER USE ALL CAPS.
- Be consistent in font, font size, and format.
- Place important words in a different color. Give your audience a tease of the topic, but they should focus on the presenter, not the slide.
- Present in the correct way to the correct audience.

(For additional guidance on PowerPoint etiquette, see http://www.muchmorebi.com/powerpoint_etiquette.htm.)

Many presenters violate these simple, basic guidelines in sharing ideas with an audience via PowerPoint. The goal is to present material in a way that you would like to see the presentation, to make a point that is memorable, and to be persuasive in what the presentation says. This usually requires a piece of content and a visual impact strategy like the PowerPoint slide example in Figure 8.5. As a nurse, you may not believe much has changed until you see a picture from another country, such as Vietnam. Figure 8.5 is a photo taken in 2005; the instructor is demonstrating how to read a mercury thermometer.

Now that you have an idea of how to present materials in a PowerPoint slide show, let's consider how to make the entire presentation an affective one.

AFFECTIVE PRESENTATION METHODS

The key to embedding affective methods into a presentation is to know what you want the group to learn. In addition, you must consider how large the group is and how they are set up in the audience. Round tables can make it easier for participants to connect in some way versus rectangular tables or just chairs in long rows. For some creative thinking on this subject, let's pick an affective outcome and look at some methods for creating the experience.

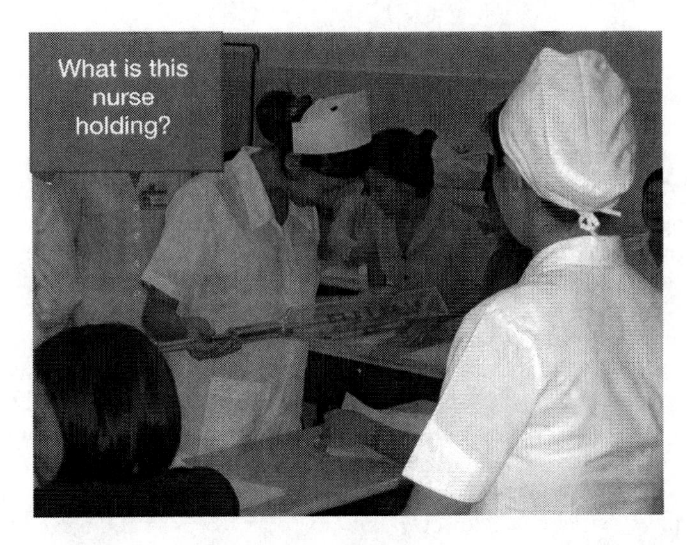

Figure 8.5 Most nurses do not see themselves as having changed their practice over time.

The subjective is: **You will have an experience of being and feeling heard.** Let's assume the worst proxemics for this presentation; that is, the room is set-up with 1,000 chairs in straight rows with spotty openings in the rows and an isle every 20 chairs across. Vignette 8.1 is a scripting of what might be accomplished toward this goal.

Vignette 8.1

I am going to give you a chance to feel what it is like to be heard. This will last for 90 seconds. First, I need all those on the aisles starting to my left—over here, you stay in place, and everyone in that row move toward that aisle person to fill in every chair. Starting to my far left, the outside person will turn to their left and touch the person closest to them on the shoulder. Continue by having the third person touch the fourth person on the shoulder, then the fourth person touches the fifth, and the fifth touches the sixth person until you each have a partner. If there is an odd number, move to a place to find a person who is also without a partner at the end of a row, but where one of you is able to touch the other person on the shoulder. Keep going until everyone has touched or been touched. We want everyone to have a partner. [Pause] Does anyone not have a partner? [You may need to match up the stragglers who may be thinking they have just escaped the process!]

Everyone can sit down, but please be slightly turned to your partner. Now, the person who did the touching is to listen. Raise your hand if you touched the other person on their shoulder. Okay, you are to LISTEN! No judgments; no "why" questions. In fact, no questions at all. You are to listen and stay tuned into your partner with your eyes and nonverbal facial cues. The person who was touched—raise your hands. Okay, you are the PRESENTERS. You will tell your partner about a trip you want to take—one that excites you. Tell them what it would mean to you to take the trip. I will ring a bell or chime in 90 seconds to indicate you must stop—now please begin.

Okay, stop! [This may take a few repeated efforts.] Now, we are going to reverse this. Those who just did the talking, raise your hands. Okay, you are to LISTEN! No judgments. No questions. Just stay present with your eyes and nonverbal facial cues. Those talking this time are to tell your partner what is in your bucket list—What is it you want to do in this life while you still can? Tell them what it would mean to you to do this. If you haven't thought of it before, well, now you can make it up. What is on your bucket list? I will ring a chime in 90 seconds for you to end—now, please begin.

Okay, stop! [Get them to stop, which may be challenging.] Listen to me for 1 minute with your eyes closed. [You may need to repeat this.] Just listen to my voice. How does it feel to be heard? How does it feel to tell someone—maybe a stranger—something that is important to you? Keep your eyes closed. If you believe this process has allowed you to feel as though you have really been heard, raise your hand. Now lower your hand, and open your eyes. [You might ask the audience to reflect in a journal for a few minutes if they have such items available.] Now I want you to tell each other how that felt for you. Take 90 seconds for both of you to say how you experienced this process. Do that now.

Okay, stop! Let's just take a quick self-assessment of your intimacy and connection scale. From a score of 1 to 10 (1 = low, 10 = high), what would you give yourself for an intimacy and connection score when you first sat down in this room? Write it down. Now, give yourself an intimacy and connection score at this very moment. Write it down. Raise your hand if you increased your score by 5 points or more.

Because of the size of this group, I cannot take questions here, but just think about this process as a way to increase your connection to others. Think about your personal sense of openness at this moment. [Pause.] Think about how you might use this process in your future. [Pause.] Assume you are a nurse, and you are about to work with some patients. Do you believe taking 90 seconds to hear your patient will have a benefit for the both of you for the next 12-hour shift together?

During a large affective experience such as this, there may be many questions that can be addressed during the reflection period for this large group. What you cannot predict is what will happen, and this often is a fear for those who need to know what will happen with each piece being presented. You are not in control of this type of process—you are facilitating an *intersubjective experience*. Many presenters would not undertake a process that they cannot control.

Different-sized groups allow for a host of presentation strategies. Smaller groups make it easier to use video clips, music, a poem, or to tell a personal story because they allow for more intimate space, closer proximity of attendees to the presenter, and it is easier for everyone to really be present to the aesthetic method being used. However, you must remember that the presentation is on a time schedule for most workshops. The more you ask participants to risk vulnerability, the more time you need to recover. In some cases, you may need to ask everyone to keep confidential anything being said in this group, but state they are allowed to talk about their own experience, just not what others have said. I have conducted one such workshop with 40 participants over two sessions of 3 hours each. This was a very impactful 6 hours with many emotions and connections that would normally never occur at a national conference.

You may be asking, "What do I have on the PowerPoint screen during these experiences?" It can be anything to calm the room or to imprint some meaning, or you can simply turn the screen off. You could be presenting on couples healing, and put up a photograph like the one below.

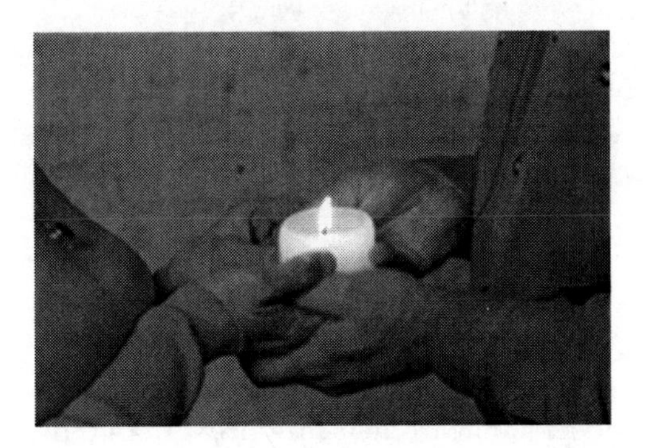

This is the time to make it impactful, but not noisy. Don't let the big screen be a distraction.

There are many strategies that can be used in a presentation that allow the group to have an affective learning experience. The initial strategy might be:

- Small groups or group breakouts
- Visualization
- Aesthetic experience (e.g., music, reading, poem, art, video, telling one's story)
- Volunteer comes to the stage to work with you
- Scripting a group of people toward one goal
- Inner and outer circles with inner circles being the work group
- A single circle of chairs if fewer than 20 people

It is not enough to have the experience; it is important to *seat* the experience in a realm of emotion regardless of what the emotion is. This is a perfect time to reinforce the affective goal presented at the beginning of the workshop. You may have had a subjective—*Create a sense of social value for the role of nurses in our community*; or, *You will have an experience of "care-in-the-moment"*—and this is the time to focus on that goal. Vignette 8.2 may be how you will structure your next presentation using objectives and subjectives.

Vignette 8.2

Topic: Today I am discussing the three types of learning in nursing practice. I will provide you with three objectives and two subjectives for your expected outcomes today.

Objectives: You will:

1. Distinguish and describe the three domains of learning
2. Analyze effective uses within each domain
3. Integrate each domain within a single class period to improve learning

Subjectives: You will experience:

1. The value of integrating the three domains
2. A sense of becoming more connected to others while learning about affective teaching

I will keep you posted on when I believe I am addressing either an objective or subjective for your learning as we discuss affective education in higher education. Let's begin.

Presentations hold many opportunities for creating affective experiences for your audience. I would not hold back on making them uncomfortable as you look to create a change in their thinking or build their self-awareness. An example of how fast it can occur is seen in Vignette 8.3.

Vignette 8.3

I want you to write on a piece of paper what color and shape a Yield traffic sign is. Do that right now. [Pause] ______________________________

Do you have it? Is your memory good? Okay, let's look.
(Play the video clip: www.trafficsign.us/yellowyield.html)

The clip shows the 20-year-old yellow yield sign and then flips to the current Yield sign that is red and white. This clip can easily move into asking those who are stuck in the past to unfreeze and think differently, because maybe they were holding onto a 20-year-old idea that yield signs are yellow. This clip can be used to illustrate how our memory cannot always be trusted and how hard it is to see anything different once we are imprinted. Affective presentations have very few limitations, but they may need some creative thinking in order to use them effectively.

SUMMARY

Presentations often need serious makeovers, and this can be done either through better use of PowerPoint slides or by adding affective content to your presentations. Take some time to think about what you would like to do the next time you present—take a risk. In doing so, you can make your presentations unforgettable.

PART III

Integrating Affective Teaching in Nursing: The Big Picture in Nursing Education

There is a string of consciousness that unifes everything and all reality. Our own filters re-interpret these things to our mind's reality, which is individual. Knowing this is called enlightenment and has been called enlightenment through the ages. (Hagelin, 2006)

CHAPTER 9

Conducting a Current Literature Review on Affective Teaching: What Does This Mean for Nursing?

> This relational way of knowing—in which love takes away fear and co-creation replaces control—is a way of knowing that can help us reclaim the capacity for connectedness on which good teaching depends. (Palmer, 2007, pp. 57–58)

In current education research around the world, educators continue to examine how affective pedagogy is impacting their students and practices. However, I have found very little discussion and current research in nursing education in this area from the past 10 years. Most of what has been written by nurse researchers comes from the mid-1990s. This does not mean we cannot learn from other disciplines conducting research on educational strategies. Therefore, in this chapter, I will look for ways to integrate recent findings from other disciplines into nursing education. Even though such integration may be hypothetical, it is useful to speculate regarding ways nursing education may begin to use current research and practice regarding affective teaching. Looking at the concepts of *emotional intelligence* (EI), e-learning, and the value of our relationships, can be powerful when considering affective teaching in nursing. This chapter examines current research on these topics and discusses ways in which we can bridge the cyclical drought that nursing education appears to be in with regard to affective teaching.

CURRENT RESEARCH USING AFFECTIVE METHODS

We examine some of the current research regarding affective teaching as an introduction to how this research may be applied to nursing education. This research comes from various fields, and in some cases includes meta-analysis regarding impacts to student learning. These recent studies do not indicate a resurgence of affective pedagogical studies on student learning outcomes. However, they do show us some ways in which current affective educational approaches have impacted other disciplines.

The first study is one by Dede (2009), which was conducted at Cumhuriye University, in Sivas, Turkey. Dede "investigated the role of comprehension tests used in teaching algebra and to examine its effects on student's success" (p. 497). One of his measurements was to examine affective competencies for these students looking at self-confidence, interest, anxiety, beliefs, motivation, and values. The comprehension testing used during this algebra course saw positive indicators by the end of the course for all six of these affective domains. Dede termed this approach *action research* and used affective measurement as an indicator of an affective teaching method. He found a correlation with improved comprehension during algebra testing using the affective competencies.

EI incorporates the idea of having self-awareness and social skills in order to be successful in certain situations life throws our way. Its utility has been examined in the field of business in particular. We examine the concept of EI in greater detail in Chapter 10. For the purposes of this chapter, however, it is worthwhile to note that EI has been considered in affective teaching, especially in K–12 settings. Thus, for this examination of current research in affective teaching, I am including a review of EI studies.

Of note is one study that challenges the belief that EI is more important than intelligence quotient (IQ) for academic success, which has been a thesis of the EI movement. Previous studies on EI's predictability of academic success were based on self-report. However, EI has been scrutinized more vigorously in recent years. Barchard (2003) conducted a study on 150 undergraduate students where he examined their cognitive domain using a "battery of 12 timed cognitive tests to measure four different first-stratum cognitive abilities" (p. 842). In addition, Barchard tested these subjects using a combination of many documented EI tests for 31 different EI measurements. He also provided some assessments on personality type to determine if these are also predictors of success. The time required for participants to complete the testing was 3.5 to 4 hours. Using multiple regression analysis, he looked to see if any of the EI domains "increased the ability to predict academic success" (p. 850). Barchard did not find any of the 31 different EI measurements able to assist faculty or students to predict their success in college. However, he did find that cognitive and personality assessments were able to predict academic success.

The work of Barchard (2003) gives some significant push-back on the value of EI attributes for better predictability of academic success, and this is worth looking at more closely. Is it possible that we need to use the broader and more recent discussion of social–emotional learning (SEL) (discussed in Chapter 10) versus the older mode of just looking at EI measurements? Regardless, consideration of what EI really is capable of offering in terms of student success will need further study, although it may not be useful for predicting academic success. However, its applications in business and leadership roles may be the key to its continued value in society. Many EI authors (discussed in Chapter 10) suggest that this is what makes a person more successful in their work life, with little said about academic success.

Turning from EI to research on teacher–student relationships, another recent examination of affective teaching concepts by Cornelius-White (2007) is of interest. In his 2007 study, he conducted a meta-analysis of the impact of a positive teacher–student relationship on learning. He examined 1,000 articles with 355,325 data points that had approximately 1,450 findings. He synthesized this huge volume of literature to 119 studies implemented from the years 1948 to 2004 and ended up with 9 independent variables and 18 dependent variables. The relationship between teacher and student has been defined as person- or learner-centered education and has also been labeled as whole-person learning using Rogerian–humanistic approaches in the classroom. Cornelius-White specifically researched six questions from the data collected to find their cumulative results for those questions. It is accepted that an $r = 0.30$ to $r = 0.33$ value would be significant at the 95% confidence level. When adding all the identified correlations, the average mean in Cornelius-White's study was $r = 0.31$. This was a significant finding for the positive value of learner-centered teaching on student outcomes.

> [The] observed confidence intervals will hold the true value of the parameter. After a sample is taken, the population parameter is either in the interval made or not, there is no chance. The desired level of confidence is set by the researcher (not determined by data). If a corresponding hypothesis test is performed, the confidence level corresponds with the level of significance, i.e., a 95% confidence interval reflects a significance level of 0.05, and the confidence interval contains the parameter values that, when tested, should not be rejected with the same sample. Greater levels of confidence give larger confidence intervals, and hence less precise estimates of the parameter. Confidence intervals of difference parameters not containing 0 imply that that there is a statistically significant difference between the populations. (Wikipedia, n.d., retrieved 10/21/12)

Cornelius-White's (2007) study showed additional significance when compared with a study by Fraser, Wahlberg, Welch, and Hattie (1987) and Hattie (1999), where they synthesized 134 meta-analyses with 7,827 studies and 5 to 15 million participants and where $r = 0.20$ for *all education strategies* used to improve student learning. These authors asserted "that any correlation greater than $r = 0.20$ is well worth pursuing, and any correlation greater than $r = 0.30$ should be of much interest." Hence, at a broad level the meta-analysis performed by Cornelius-White showed that "learner-centered relationships are well worth pursuing" (Cornelius-White, p. 130).

When Cornelius-White (2007) specifically examined affective and behavioral outcomes, he found significant correlations between participation and initiation with learner-centered pedagogy with an $r = 0.55$. There were additional positive correlations with student motivation ($r = 0.32$) and student satisfaction ($r = 0.44$). He also found a correlation to a reduction in dropouts ($r = 0.35$) and a reduction in disruptive behavior and absences ($r = 0.25$).

In addition to testing a particular teaching method, some have studied student learning styles and how these might impact acceptance of certain teaching methods to include affective pedagogy. Mather and Champagne (2008) discussed how complex this subject is, as most faculty in higher education are not educated formally as teachers. Mather and Champagne's study explored the impact of learning styles combined with a teacher's pedagogy and its impact on learning. Mather and Champagne referenced research that showed learning styles affect comprehension, classroom performance, study strategies, and test-taking techniques, and they explored specific learning styles and how these students interpreted what they read.

Mather and Champagne (2008) studied undergraduates at the University of Lethbridge who were in their third year of college. They studied 436 students in health sciences, social sciences, management, and science courses. The authors examined ten courses from each of these four areas, and six trained independent faculty examined the courses for learning–teaching strategies. The students were assessed for learning styles, and then the researchers correlated student's perceptions of the learning methods provided during the classes they completed. These authors found that student learning was genuinely heterogeneous with themes found with certain groups of students. These authors identified that science students do not typically value feeling and intuitive pedagogy (affective pedagogy). The science students were primarily male; however, both males and females had similar results if they were science majors. Education and engineering faculty almost exclusively preferred to teach using clear organized lecturing format with minimal affective methods. This study was very confusing in its conclusions, but what was evident is that students' styles vary dramatically and teachers tend to use what they know regardless of what would best serve the student. Faculty do not vary their teaching methods for the types of students in the classroom. In addition, a warning to students is suggested by these authors, where there is little value in knowing your learning style unless faculty consider varying their pedagogy based on the class mix (Cuthbert, 2005).

Very little research is being conducted presently on affective teaching or on its use as a measurement for an outcome involving teaching methods. It is unfortunate, but there has been an obvious slowing after the heavy focus found in the mid-1990s. Although not mentioned as a cause for this phenomenon, there may be a waning process regarding the value of separating learning into cognitive and affective domains, as suggested in earlier chapters. Whatever the reason, we are not seeing any resurgence of affective pedagogical studies on student learning outcomes.

Affective Teaching and EI Impact on Nursing

Chapter 10 is dedicated to the impact of EI and SEL on nursing affective pedagogy and effective teaching and provides an excellent summary of its value stemming from Palmer's work. For this chapter, however, it is useful to have a brief introduction to the value of EI and SEL in nursing education. Palmer (2007) called using such teacher self-awareness and regulation as *good teaching* and identifies the following as characteristics of good teaching:

- A capacity to combine structure or intentionality with flexibility in both planning and leading the class: clarity about the objectives but openness to various ways of achieving them
- Thorough knowledge of the material assigned to the students and a commitment to helping them master that material
- A desire to help the students build a bridge between the academic text and their own lives and a strategic approach for doing so
- A respect for students' stories that is no more or less than the respect for the scholarly texts assigned to them
- An ability to see students' lives more clearly than they themselves see them, a capacity to look beyond their initial self-presentation, and a desire to help them see themselves more deeply
- An aptitude for asking good questions and listening carefully to students' responses—not only to what they say but also to what they leave unsaid
- A willingness to take risks, especially the risk of inviting open dialogue, since one can never know where it is going to take us (pp. 71–72)

Palmer's characteristics allow us to correlate effective teaching, SEL goals, and what some might consider to be exceptional teachers. Please refer to Chapter 10 for more detail on this correlation.

E-LEARNING AND AFFECTIVE PEDAGOGY

Bernard et al. (2009) conducted a meta-analysis on three different types of distance learning (e-learning) and analyzed 74 studies for:

1. Student–student interaction
2. Student–teacher interaction
3. Student–content interaction

The authors gained some insights as they reviewed the literature to include the problem of comparing distance education to classroom instruction. Such comparisons take away from a deeper assessment of what is useful for just improving distance education alone. They determined that classroom instruction best practices do not translate well to distance learning best practices, and this comparison between distance and in-seat education has been the focus of most distance learning research.

In addition, the authors found that there are examples of distance education that are better than and worse than classroom instruction methods for increasing student achievement. The two distance educational strategies included in the analysis were asynchronous (mostly correspondence and online) and synchronous (mostly teleconferencing and satellite based). The authors found asynchronous was more often superior to classroom instruction in terms of achievement and student attitudes about the course. However, asynchronous distance education has more challenges with course completion. This certainly would suggest the need for additional research on what constitutes quality achievement for e-learning courses. In my own experience, I also see higher grades for e-learning courses versus classroom instruction, but I believe there is a serious shortcoming in how we assess learning for e-learning courses as well as compare the two methods related to long-term knowledge retention.

From an affective experience perspective, Bernard et al. (2009) found studies that support the need for student–student interaction and student–teacher synchronous or a blended distance educational experience in order to have positive affective student experiences. The authors believe there is a social presence and personal satisfaction that is derived from these live connections. The overall study results suggest that student–teacher interactions "are less effective, possibly more difficult to implement consistently, or provide less added value than student–student or student–content interactions" (p. 1259). The second result "suggests that increasing the strength of interaction treatments affects achievement" in a positive way (p. 1260). This seems to be true for any form of distance education. This would also be supported by theories on relational-centered or learner-centered teaching as being valuable to improve student achievement.

The third result of this affective distance education study "suggests that stronger student–content interaction treatments provide achievement advantages over weaker student–content interaction treatments" (Bernard et al., 2009, p. 1260). This may seem obvious and brings up the question why the authors even examined this issue. The fourth result suggests "the combination of student–student plus student–teacher [interactions] was not significant" (p. 1261) for improving student achievement. This seems to be borne out by the next result, as it invalidates our preconceived notions regarding better distance education using combined methods. The fifth question was to assess the difference between the asynchronous and synchronous versus mixed forms of distance education. The idea of mixing methods has been seen as more effective by Bernard et al., but this was not validated by the data analysis. There does not seem to be any advantage in mixing methods. Their study does not offer much insight into how an affective experience might be created during distance education, but the potential is there for synchronous methods that experiment with strategies for improving the relationship between the students or between the student and the instructor.

Imagine a teaching method that shows some humanism during the interactions, an open dialogue asking for critical reflection on issues of power, or preconceived assumptions versus posttreatment assumptions. This study does help clarify that quality teaching needs to be present either in distance education or classroom instruction. Both are at risk for lacking in affective pedagogy and potentially having teachers who would be labeled as traditional or surface teachers.

Shen, Wang, and Shen (2009) studied how to improve e-learning using emotion feedback to correct the misperceptions of the e-learning content. They believed e-learning should generate positive learning achievements and also improve student engagement in the learning process if the content could have an immediate correction based on the instructor knowing the emotions being generated by the student. These authors were interested in determining if adding an emotional content feedback correction would improve learner outcomes. There are a few significant issues that present themselves in this study. The first is the technique of measuring affective–biological (emotion) data (e.g., heart rate, skin conduction, electroencephalography [EEG], and blood pressure using finger electrodes). The more serious question is their use of one subject being tested over a week and collecting 43,200 data points. Certainly such an approach risks generalizability, but probably it gives the reader some idea of the effect of the process for this one student. The most common emotion during the experiment was confusion that was quickly turned into engagement when the e-learning module operators were able to see the emotional response of the student. The emotional correction method was 91% more effective in promoting learning than the method of not providing corrections for emotional responses. However, it is hard to imagine how this can be effectively conducted on more than one subject and then compare the findings. This was such an extensive study on an $N = 1$ that it seems impossible to conduct these measurements on a substantially larger number of subjects.

Assessing a student's emotional response to some learning event may seem to be impractical. However, this may be what is happening when excellent teachers intuitively assess for emotions such as frustration or confusion in a classroom, and then make corrections in the moment or for the next session for improved learning. It would be ideal to say that *affective teachers* are those who have their emotional antennae out in order to catch the collective emotion of the class and then make subtle changes that are smooth, nonshaming, and offer clarification to what is being discussed. Maybe the clarification comes in the form of a personal experience that represents the issues using thick description and storytelling—two very useful affective strategies. This would be much more difficult to assess in a typical e-learning or distance education process. It might be something for future assessments of students' emotional tone to have a skin conductor attached to every computer used for an online class. The instructor could receive a collective stress response graph as the discussion continued and then could make emotional corrections online—or maybe even in the classroom. However, it is likely we will continue to make these adjustments this intuitively, especially with emotionally intelligent literate faculty looking for signals that suggest something is wrong.

Impact on Affective Teaching in Nursing From e-Learning Research

So what can we take away from the e-learning research outlined above with regard to nursing education? Nursing education continues to grow additional distance learning methods that are synchronous and asynchronous. The studies discussed suggest we have more to learn about what has been working and what makes no difference or detracts from e-learning. Researchers have found teaching practices that are better than and worse than e-learning methods. The information presented may also advise us on some of the best ways to mix our teaching methods without trying to move to higher levels of synchronous teaching in nursing. There are students who do better on their own and in their own time frame using asynchronous methods but we don't know if we are assessing long-term learning using any of these methods.

There have been studies conducted on the use of emotion as a corrective feedback method, and we learned about measuring emotional responses in students. I believe there is potential in these studies for nursing, but more than likely, nursing education will remain relatively intuitive in such feedback for some time to come.

RELATIONAL EDUCATION

In our examination of current literature and its impacts on affective teaching in nursing, it is useful to consider what has been termed relational education. Relational education is founded in certain beliefs. Bingham and Sidorkin (2004) suggest educators consider the following propositions:

1. A relation is more real than the things it brings together. Human beings and nonhuman things acquire reality only in relation to other beings and things.
2. The self is a knot in the web of multiple intersecting relations; pull relations out of the web, and you will not find self. We do not have relations; relations have us.
3. Authority and knowledge are not something one has, but relationships are what requires others to enact.
4. Human relations exist in and through shared practices.

5. Relations are complex: They may not be described in single utterances. To describe a relation is to produce a multivoiced text.
6. Relations are primary; actions are secondary. Human words and actions have no authentic meaning; they acquire meaning only in a context of specific relations.
7. Teaching is building educational relations. Aims of teaching and outcomes of learning can both be defined as specific forms of relations to oneself, people around the students, and the larger world.
8. Educational relation is different from any other; its nature is transitional. Educational relation exists to include the student in a wider web of relations beyond the limits of the educational relation.
9. Relations are not necessarily good; human relationality is not an ethical value. Domination is as relational as love. (pp. 6–7)

We can build upon these relational beliefs by considering the value of any relationship, especially as they relate to the relationships between students and teachers. Halldorsdottir (1991) created a model for measuring a relationship's value and Watson (2008) expanded upon this model. Halldorsdottir and Watson's models outline a value scale for relationships. At the first level is *biocidic*, which is defined as life destroying. It is toxic to those around you and is full of anger, despair, and may even cause disease. It has been called *vampire energy* (Slate, 2002) that can even reshape auras and can impact the crystallization of frozen water (Emoto, 2004) by distorting the molecules so they cannot form nice symmetrical patterns. A discussion of the research by Emoto is found at www.youtube.com/watch?v=33IiYb8htHk&feature=youtu.be. The second level is *biostatic*, which is life restraining. We see this in someone with a cold or confrontational demeanor who seems to see anything outside the self as a nuisance. The third is *biopassive* and is called life neutral. At this level of connection you may think it is acceptable because we are exposed to so many of these neutral and detached persons, but these authors suggest it is a dangerous relational state. To be detached from those you are teaching or caring for is not a health-supporting connection. The fourth is *bioactive* and is called life sustaining. In this place we see a positive connection develop and the relationship is kind, concerned, and benevolent. A teacher in this type of relationship is someone who does many of the immediacy and care pedagogy verbal and nonverbal behaviors identified earlier. Students will know when teachers are connecting at this level. The last relational state is *biogenic* and is considered life giving and life receiving. Faculty who work from this domain have a significant level of self-awareness, are calm, and are not triggered by events in the classroom while still managing the dynamics of the different personalities in the room as well as the topic at hand. They function on multiple levels in order to understand what they are hearing and can make personal changes in the moment to address what they are learning and how they are teaching the topic at hand. The face of a biogenic teacher might appear as calm and beatific as Yoda (from *Star Wars*), Gandhi, or biblical prophets—and yes, you may be one of these teachers.

> Good teachers possess a capacity for connectedness. They are able to weave a complex web of connections among themselves, their subjects, and their students so that students can learn to weave a world for themselves. The methods used by these weavers vary widely: lectures, Socratic dialogue, laboratory experiments, collaborative problem solving, creative chaos. The connections made by good teachers are held not in their methods but in their hearts—meaning heart in the ancient sense, as the place where intellect and emotion and spirit will converge in the human self. (Palmer, 2007, p. 11)

Let's consider how patients might perceive the various relationship levels by reading about the experience in Vignette 9.1.

Vignette 9.1

Laura Hays, a nurse of 29 years who was close to death from septic shock in 2008, presents her experience in a poem. She presents herself from her ICU bed where she believes she is facing death. Later, Laura was able to experience and reflect on all types of relationships that occurred during her dying moments—sometimes more conscious than other times. She later wrote:

The "Eyes" Have It . . . The Caring Moment: One Nurse to Another

One nurse lied to another that I had refused to be catheterized suggesting me a "difficult patient," my care compromised I was a change of shift transfer, I vulnerably realized . . . .

One nurse is clearly a memory of his back turned or silent stare, his lack of presence loud in my isolation of intensive care. I can't recall his humanness to validate existence in his lair . . . .

Another talked at me of the virtues of getting up while task-like changing my sheet, "You need to prevent crumbs in bed to feel better," her advice complete. Never discovering death still clutched my mind and life an uncertain feat. Never asking my perspective that even crumbs in my bed would be sweet . . . .

However, I am grateful for Caritas Healers. Two students and their mentor brought me smiles, time, and laughter touching my recovery with light, healing me much faster. I wept fearing discharge and experienced compassion after . . . .

A housekeeper partook of my lavender lotion with unabashed pleasure. Joining my world with delight; uplifting many patients with great measure; reminding my husband and me of simple interactions hold an incredible treasure . . . .

And one nurse in particular is etched in my semi-conscious memory; her eyes burning through my glassy black sight with Love expressed sagely searching for who and where I lived inside; knowing death perched ready for me.

I remember her eyes called with Authentic Presence as a mother for her child; come back so I of may know you; Mindful your Life is not yet filed.

She honored Nightingale and me, touching sacredly, reflectively;
For hours she labored without complaint, her heart shown radiantly.

Intense, complex, moving faster and faster, change IV orders on-a-dime.
My mind held the intentional connection her eyes first revealed fine;

Ethically Holding Life more than I at that disrupted darkened Time;
Forever touching my Soul, she has become a quiet History of mine . . .

—Laura Hayes (2010)

Vignette 9.1 outlines how a nurse-patient perceived the various relationships she experienced in this real-life situation. This would be a powerful teaching tool for students, but it also has importance in the self-evaluation of our teaching methods. Consider the type of teacher you are. What kind of relationship do you want to have with your students? And how can you get there if you are not there already? The following discussion examines how we can build relationships by providing some insights into how to use tension to create self-awareness and learning.

Creating Inner Tension Creates Self-Awareness

Mayo (2004) suggests that students need to have their habits broken in order to begin "thinking and acting differently, . . . having to face and understand an obstacle in order to stop and think" (p. 122). She suggests there is value in mixing up comfortable groups to create new tension to support self-awareness. There is a need to get uncomfortable in order to learn and to build new relationships. Relationships are difficult and students need to practice what it takes to start one and maintain it. "As much as obstacles pull the learner into a realization of ignorance, the *apora* [what centers you] is filled, eventually, by what the learner already knew in the otherworld" (p. 125). Students and faculty members need to battle their own inner shaping that came from their family and cultural development in order to build a relationship. This is not easy.

Nodding (2005) sees the caring relationship at the core of affective teaching. It is what teachers create as they show care or "engrossment," which is a type of care in which the teacher empties his or her own content in order to let the student give feedback to the teacher who is fully "receptive" (p. 16). Nodding also challenges the notion that knowledge can affect this type of relationship:

> We suppose that knowledge will reduce misunderstanding, stereotyping, and the almost instinctive fear of strangers. But knowledge alone is unlikely to establish caring relations. In fact, a number of studies have shown that qualities such as "counselor relationship"

> or "teacher relationship" are only slightly correlated with multicultural knowledge. Knowing something about other cultures is important and useful, but it is not sufficient to produce positive relationships. (p. 113)

Nodding has been at the center of this type of educational reform for many years, and certainly would be in excellent company within nursing education.

Some question the value or appropriateness of building strong relationships in the academic setting. Thayer-Bacon (2004) disagrees with Nodding's description of student–teacher relationships and would certainly disagree with what has been presented earlier related to presence, care pedagogy, and teaching as an expression of love. She believes United States society makes significant distinctions and supports a separation between private and public relations. She would support a more neutral relationship that has been termed *biostatic*. There may be good legal reasons to keep a more *biostatic* relationship, but it certainly impacts what the students will learn or not learn based on what has been described in this chapter. In addition, McDaniel (2004) believes that we need to ask, "Can relationships be harmful as well as nurturing?" (p. 91). He actually begs the question, as he is concerned with how caring relationships in the public world might cloud rather than promote a deeper and more intellectual discussion. He quotes Eamonn Callan who wrote *Creating Citizens* (2004/1997) by stating, "It is better to conceptualize citizens' moral dialogue as occurring among detached strangers, rather than soul mates" (p. 92).

This detachment behavior has been the traditional and accepted thought in education, nursing, and medicine for hundreds of years. Nursing has been more likely to break this tradition, but nursing still has large pockets where faculty teach *professional detachment*. Today, we continue this debate and hear the concern but may wonder if this is what is needed or is this reflective of the comfort zone of the faculty and students who support this view. For the sake of affective literacy in our students, I am hopeful we will continue to embrace the relational classroom using the principles of Nodding (2005), Palmer (2007), and Watson (2008).

Relational Teaching for Nursing

> There is an intimacy about it in the sense that I'm not so sure that in a face-to-face encounter we are really, truly able to transmit teaching to those who we do not love. (Hooks, 1999, p. 125)

The discussion of relational-teaching and how it supports learning-centered classrooms is a key issue for *affective teaching*. It builds on the intersubjective knowing and the philosophy of teaching the whole person. There is significant application of *care and immediacy* pedagogy as a way to address relational teaching. It is almost self-evident how valuable this research is to the thesis of this text.

SUMMARY

There seems to have been a shift after the year 2000 to a lack of interest in investigating either curricula or teaching methods that focus on affective teaching methods. We have started to see some movement in the world of e-learning, but it is still significantly lacking in terms of how educators might use affective teaching methods or if they are desirable in distance learning. This reduced attention to the affective domain of education is reminiscent of how cyclical we are in education and specifically nursing education, where we move in and out of various topics. There are times when we have heavy, thunderous emphasis on a certain academic strategy that is then followed by a drought. It seems we are currently in such a drought period when it comes to affective teaching.

However, the support for relational educational methods and learner-centered classrooms continues and is supported within and outside of nursing education. The academic voices from the 1980s and 1990s continue to advocate for our educational system to change. They want our teaching to be based on caring relationships that continue to reject *biostatic* and detached approaches to our students. Several have questioned if the academic setting is the place for a relational experience; others are emphatic that we must have it to be effective educators. "There is an intimacy about it in the sense that I'm not so sure that in a face-to-face encounter we are really, truly able to transmit teaching to those who we do not love" (Hooks, 1999, p. 125). I would also suggest that this might be true by the way we respond within distance learning. We continually need to show our love to our students, regardless of the medium we are using.

CHAPTER 10

The Emotional and Social Intelligence Movement

HISTORICAL DEVELOPMENT OF SOCIAL–EMOTIONAL LEARNING

The *emotional intelligence (EI)* movement started to gain strength in the early to mid-1990s. In later years, authors started to integrate social intelligence into their writing on EI, which became the *social–emotional learning (SEL)* movement. To understand the historical relevance to our discussion of affective literacy, it is important to note that there are prolific SEL works that started in the business world (Boyatzis & Van Oosten, 2002; Cherniss, 2000; Cherniss & Goleman, 1998; Cooper, 1997; Goleman, 1998, 1995; Weisinger, 1997) and have now flourished in the world of education (Cohen, 2001; Elias, 2009, 2006; Elias et al., 1997; Hoffman, 2009; Goleman, 2006; Graczyk, et al., 2000; Steiner, 1997; Zins, Weissberg, Wang, & Walberg, 2004, to name a few). Educators have provided many strategies for the idea of EI since it first appeared in print by Salovey and Mayer in 1990. It only took a few years for investigators to see parallels with EI constructs and those found in social competency programs in education even prior to 1990 (Rotheram-Boris & Tsembaris, 1989).

> Ostensibly, the SEL [social–emotional learning] movement is about changing educational practice in ways that support positive emotional climates in classrooms and schools by building individual emotional competencies. (Hoffman, 2009, p. 548)

The term *emotional literacy* goes back further to the 1970s when the clinical psychologist Claude Steiner defined it as "the ability to understand your emotions, the ability to listen to others and empathize with their emotions, and the ability to express emotions productively" (Steiner, 1997, p. 11). Goleman's (1995) definition of EI was "being able to rein in emotional impulse; to read another's innermost feelings; to handle relationships smoothly" (p. xiii). This definition was later changed to: "emotional intelligence is the capacity for recognizing our own feelings and those of others, for motivating ourselves, and for managing emotions well in ourselves and in our relationships" (1998, p. 317). Goleman's (1998) adaptation included EI and social intelligence (SI) domains, which were self-awareness, self-regulation, motivation, empathy, and social skills. (A video clip of Daniel Goleman presenting his theory nationally can be viewed at http://www.youtube.com/watch?v=Y7m9eNoB3NU&feature=youtu.be.) A more recent definition of EI is:

> Emotional intelligence is observed when a person demonstrates the competencies that constitute self-awareness, self-management, social awareness, and social skills at appropriate times and ways in sufficient frequency to be effective in situations. (Boyatzis, Goleman, & Rhee, 1999, p. 343)

This seems to be a useful working definition for many settings, although the reason EI and SEL are being discussed in this text on affective teaching may not be evident. Let's compare the above definition with our working definition of affective pedagogy found in Chapter 1, which is a teaching method that is:

> A form of teaching that will support the individual's integration of knowledge regarding emotion, preference, choice, feeling, belief, attitude, ethic, and personal awareness of the self.

One might expect that the EI and SEL movements might have been more inclusive of the affective teaching and learning domains, but it seems they were rarely integrated. However, they are significantly related, as presented in the following.

SEL FOR HIGHER EDUCATION

Most of the SEL educational models and research are used in K–12 settings where there is a need to instill competencies and skill development for young children and young adults as a way to improve socialization abilities. There is some research on using these skills in adult classrooms so teachers and students learn to work together more effectively. Such work is closely tied to affective literacy for teachers and social–emotional literacy for both teachers and students. However, there is also a significant cognitive component to how SEL is being used in many settings. For example, Hoffman (2009) identified several purely cognitive models in practice that are aimed at producing measurable outcomes for students learning SEL. He states:

> The emphasis on emotional skills reveals that emotion per se is not the focus; rather, it is the cognitive processing of emotion that is important—the "reasoning about" emotion and the behaviors one associated with such reasoning. SEL is fundamentally about psychometric and pedagogical possibility: Skills can be taught and the learner's competence in their performance can be measured. (p. 538)

This emphasis on skill and cognitive processing of emotions has been seen as a valuable outcome for successful SEL training of students going into the world of life and work (Cohen, 2006; Goleman, 1995; Stern, 2007).

Of greater concern in this review of SEL is how teachers might use, model, and mentor such skills as proof of its value in the classroom, if they do use such strategies. A video clip of a national speaker who uses SEL for teaching acceptance in grade schools is available at www.youtube.com/watch?v=XfyC0o88zfM&feature=youtu.be. Hoffman's (2009) research and essay on the subject present a serious problem in this area, stating:

> Many SEL programs similarly highlight the key role of empathetic, caring, supportive relationships among teachers, students, and parents; cooperative learning opportunities; and allowing students both autonomy and influence in the classroom. . . . However, the caring community, when translated into practice, becomes a discourse about activities and behaviors. . . . In effect, substance is replaced by structure; feeling is replaced by form. Most tellingly, caring and community are conceptualized as things teachers teach children to do by getting them to behave in appropriate ways. (p. 545)

> Good teaching cannot be reduced to technique; good teaching comes from the identity and integrity of the teacher. (Palmer, 2007, p. 10)

Faculty who are teaching adults have an even greater challenge. The students in the classroom have already formed many opinions regarding education, their need to learn (or not), whether the instructor is a good teacher (or not), and may have a host of reasons for being in that course, ranging from an excitement about learning to a boredom that is tied to simply taking a required course for their major. No longer are you dealing with SEL as a proper way to ask for help on an assignment. Even in K–12, this becomes a technique to teach rather than a community norm of activity based on Hoffman's research. Palmer (2007) puts it this way: "Good teaching cannot be reduced to technique; good teaching comes from the identity and integrity of the teacher" (p. 10). He relates this to knowing yourself as a teacher and that you are "willing to make it available and vulnerable in the service of learning" (p. 11).

SEL in higher education can take lessons from what we have been seeing for 20 years in K–12; we must still heed the caution from experts in these programs:

> I am a bit bothered by the great emphasis in current research on teaching the kids social skills such as listening. Of course it is important for students to learn how to listen and treat one another with come sensitivity, but it is also important that teachers listen to the students. (Nodding, 2006, p. 239)

It is therefore important to integrate the "identity and integrity of the teacher" as noted by Palmer (2007, p. 10) with the socialization and the cognitive emotional processing by the student. For effective and full implementation of SEL, such a student–teacher partnership is truly a two-way street.

How we implement SEL may be further examined by breaking it down into smaller segments and examining each in the learning environment. Goleman (1998) presents the following five clusters for SEL:

1. Self-awareness cluster
2. Self-regulation cluster
3. Motivation cluster
4. Empathy cluster
5. Social skills cluster

What would it look like to see faculty in a nursing program address the five clusters for SEL presented by Goleman? To do this, let's examine what each of these means and how their usefulness may be applied in an academic setting in various ways using vignettes. These vignettes are taken from a group process that has been used in mental health classes to help students and patients heal. This method is highly affective in nature and can create life changes in the students who use this process.

Self-Awareness Cluster

This includes emotional awareness, accurate self-assessment, and self-confidence.

Vignette 10.1 describes an entire day of self-awareness strategies using letter writing. It could be broken out over many sessions or could be used for a day-long workshop.

Vignette 10.1

Hi, faculty. It is good to see you today. We will be spending the morning working on our self-awareness, assessing what we can do and what we are challenged to do for our own self-growth and building some self-confidence by looking at ways to be successful in this challenging area of EI. Jean Watson (2008) explores a complete process of becoming a caring nurse through the Caritas Nursing experience and this includes our need to be in touch with our humanity. So today we will be working on our ability to address four key human needs. Let's start by taking out a pad of paper and pen. At the top of the first page, write "forgiveness." Now here is what you will be doing for the next 20 minutes:

- ***Forgiveness:*** Write a short letter (no names) to someone in your life who has done something that you have never been able to forgive. Think of this person in the broader sense that he or she has a hook in you that needs to be removed. The hook is your energy in hanging on to being angry with whatever he or she did. This person put the hook in you, and for some reason it is still there. Now imagine taking that hook out of your skin—the hook represents your anger and pain about what happened. Give the hook back to that person in this letter you are writing, and if possible, tell the person you forgive him or her for how he or she treated you—it was not okay, but the person did it, and you have been angry ever since that time. Explain that it was unfortunate that this is how that person needed to be with you, but you forgive him or her for being so misguided.

  If this is too difficult, then forgive yourself for leaving the hook of pain and anger in your flesh all this time, and picture yourself taking it out and then let it go. Give it back to the person who put it there and say, "This is yours. I no longer need it. I have learned that it no longer serves me to keep it in my flesh. You can have it back and thanks for showing me that I don't need this pain and anger to be okay any longer." Take 20 minutes to write your letter. Go outside, sit under a tree, but don't talk to anyone else while doing this piece. It is private—for only you. It is your Forgiveness letter. Return in 20 minutes.
- ***Offering Gratitude***: On a separate sheet of paper, write the name of someone who did something for you for which you have gratitude. He or she gave you something special in your life. He or she may be living or may have passed away, but you really never told this person how much you appreciate what he or she did or how he or she was present in your life. You are going to write a letter to this person. This letter is one that you might mail; you might just call and tell him or her what you have written; you may need to bury the letter at the grave site after reading it; or you may read it to others because the person is no longer living. In any case, write the letter and take the next 20 minutes in a place of solitude to contemplate your gratitude for him or her.
- ***Surrender***: Surrender brings up many issues for people, and I realize that many of the immediate responses seem very negative and you have no desire to go there—such as surrendering and losing yourself, and so forth. That is not what this is. I want you to think of a child who surrenders to your affection and then hugs you with a complete openness to being loved. So take out a piece of paper and at the top, write down the word "surrender" or "surrender with love." Is there someone or something in your life that you need to surrender to in a way that allows you to let go of a part that no longer serves you? It could be that someone is attempting to be very affectionate with you, but you push back; you want the students to all "get it" and not all of them do; you feel the need for control of all the interactions in the classroom but can't get it done; you must be perfect in your teaching and can't seem to get there; your children demand your time when you get home from work, and you feel you have no energy to give them. Pick one thing you believe you can surrender to and let go of your current pattern for dealing with it. Write that down now.

You will take 20 minutes to thank that part of you that has hung on so desperately to this behavior. It was attempting to serve you in some way, but it no longer is working. Now say that you surrender to what needs to happen next—to your next and new step for this issue in your life. Write it clearly, "I surrender my _____, and am willing to let what I really want to happen in this situation take its place." Find a place of solitude and write, and then return in 20 minutes.

- ***Overcoming Fear and Pride***: You may not believe the power of fear in our lives today; however, it has been described by Don Miguel Ruiz (1999) as the disease of humanity that is so prevalent that we don't know it is still our greatest disease. In fact, it is so common that we don't even think of it as a disease any longer. In the world of the teacher, Parker Palmer (2007) provided several areas that hold fear for faculty: fear of the student being him/herself; fear of connection; fear of conflict; fear of losing one's identity; and fear of transformational change. He presents the discussion of Jan Tompkin (1991) who states: "Fear of showing up for what you are: a fraud, stupid, ignorant, a clod, a dolt, a sap, a weakling, someone who can't cut the mustard" (in Palmer, p. 30).

  Closely related to this is the mask teachers wear in order to deal with their fear—the mask of pride. This is a pride built around the inauthentic self. Where is it that you overcompensate or find yourself vulnerable to being embarrassed by making a mistake in class; in giving an assignment inaccurately? Both fear and pride come from our inability to be authentic teachers, to include the vulnerability that comes with being authentic. Write at the top of your paper the words Fear and Pride. I want you to spend time on both of these as much as you can in 30 minutes. Maybe give 15 minutes to each. For the fear area, write down your greatest fears about your teaching—what is it you would dread any person knowing about what you are thinking, how you struggle with core issues that you may feel could destroy your career? Then take some time to look at how you compensate for this fear. How does pride or any inauthentic behavior help you cope with this fear of being found out? Find a place of solitude to write. It is time to find the dark places that you hide, repress, and deny. See you in 30 minutes.
- ***Integration and Self-Awareness:*** We are going to sit in a circle to discuss what we are learning about our teaching and ourselves using some rules by Parker Palmer (2004). Only one person can speak at a time. Do not respond to another person's comments with a fix; in this exercise, there is no saving or reassuring, and no advice-giving. You can only speak for yourself, so use "I" statements. Give your name, say what is important to you, and end with a statement about what you are learning about yourself. The comment from the group will be—"Thank you for sharing." We will end in 60 minutes, so take a risk and say what you need to say.

Self-awareness is not easy, and there have been no publications or research on ways of making this process easy. Creating a "Caritas Consciousness" (Watson, 2008, p. 232) is certainly a demanding process that is described in much more detail by the authors of *Shadow Work*, or *Inner Growth Work* (Dayton, 1994; Deci & Flaste, 1995; Downing, 1991; Ford, 2002; Napier, 1990). Given the demanding nature of understanding self-awareness and the relative lack of guidance on how to make this easier, is there any wonder why

Hoffman (2009) sees only a cognitive or process approach to SEL activities in the classroom? It is much easier to focus on the students' SEL skill building rather than partnering with them and exposing a teacher's own vulnerability in order to achieve the heightened level of self-awareness that is required for true SEL in education. Consider this statement:

> It is not simply a matter of teaching students' topics and skills associated with social and emotional learning. It is essentially a matter of showing, by our own acts and attitudes, that we care about what students (teachers) are going through and that we are partners in the search for meaning. (Nodding, 2006, p. 240)

The next section examines the next cluster in SEL as outlined by Goleman (1998)—self-regulation.

Self-Regulation Cluster

This includes self-control, trustworthiness, conscientiousness, adaptability, and innovation.

To self-regulate requires many inner attributes that can be adapted and build trust. Vignette 10.2 provides an example of an instructor who is willing to partner with a class in order to have the maximum learning integration of gifts from the students and the teacher to achieve self-regulation.

Vignette 10.2

Teacher: I am looking for a way that we can create a new way of being in the classroom that supports your needs and mine. You may be thinking that it is my job as the teacher to create this. However, I am proposing that since this is our first class together, we can create something unique where all of us participate in the process. The goal would be that we create a class self-regulation process, and each one of us can ask for more or less regulation as we move through the course together. Yes, I have experience with what has or has not worked well in the past, and I have approximately 8 years' experience teaching the content of Nursing Research with other groups similar to yours as well as at the master's level. What I don't have is your knowledge, experience, fears, or understanding of research and how you want it to fit into your life as a nurse.

In front of you is the course syllabus that tells you everything we are being asked to cover regarding this topic. What it does not say is how most nurses are using this knowledge in their careers as front-line nurses. In addition, the syllabus does not say why so many let all this knowledge slip away soon after they leave the course. Within the syllabus, you will see that I am asked by the college to ensure you know certain aspects related to research. Some of this is terminology, but the greatest sharing would be to assist you to integrate your knowledge of formal inquiry methods, to look at what it means to have scientific rigor, and to read what others have published in the name of research and see if you can critique their work in a way to make it meaningful for your practice and what type of feedback you would give them if they were in the room with us.

Let's start this discussion by looking at the course content outline and check everything that is new to you. Then let's look at the text to see where you can read about most of the issues you have checked and how much of that material you would like me to assist you with during the course using some lecture and discussion strategies.

Next, are you curious about things you have read already, and/or would you like me to bring in research that I find challenging to address in our current nursing work environment? We can do both, but let's do it in teams of five or six students so we can create some discussions on the topics and let the others hear our discussions. Maybe they have insights after hearing the small group discuss the study. Would that work for you? If you have a study you want to review, bring six copies of it next week to class.

How are you all doing with process? Any concerns so far that we should discuss?

Student: What about the testing on the syllabus? It says we have three quizzes and two exams with a comprehensive final.

Teacher: Yes, it does. It even has percentages attached to these along with a grade for one written critique. So—imagine this is also your class and my class. I need to know what you know at the end. If my only parameter is that you can integrate ideas from your text, from the things you want me to teach you in class, and from our own practice with looking and critiquing research in class to include our discussions, then tell me how you would like to get a grade for what you have done, and what grade you would get if you could only do some of what I want at the end? Any ideas—and all ideas—are okay to put on the board. We only have to agree on what we will do at the end of this discussion.

Every new course requires a review of what is expected as objectives, hopefully subjectives, content outline, learning outcomes, grading strategy, sometimes what is expected of students and faculty, rubrics used to objectify more subjective activities, and references to be used to include required readings. As a teacher practicing the second cluster of EI, things might look very different. The use of *intersubjectivity* comes into play as a way of being with your students, and a way for the teacher to learn. Goleman (2006) presents this as a "meshing of two people's inner worlds" (p. 107). The idea was called *unknowing* by Munhall (1993) as two or more people created a new reality in the moment. Palmer (2007) called using such teacher self-awareness and regulation as *good teaching* and identifies the following characteristics of this *intersubjectivity* (also mentioned in Chapter 9):

- A capacity to combine structure or intentionality with flexibility in both planning and leading the class; clarity about the objectives but openness to various ways of achieving them
- Thorough knowledge of the material assigned to students and a commitment to helping them master that material
- A desire to help students build a bridge between the academic text and their own lives as well as a strategic approach for doing so
- A respect for students' stories that is no more or less than the respect for the scholarly texts assigned to them
- An ability to see students' lives more clearly than they themselves see them, a capacity to look beyond their initial self-presentation, and a desire to help them see themselves more deeply
- An aptitude for asking good questions and listening carefully to students' responses—not only to what they say, but also to what they leave unsaid
- A willingness to take risks, especially the risk of inviting open dialogue, though we can never know where it is going to take us (pp. 71–72)

It is easy to see a correlation between SEL domains and the practice of being an effective and balanced teacher—maybe even an *exceptional teacher.*

The third cluster for this new EI or SEL involves motivation. What is it that motivates us as teachers, and can we stimulate our motivation when needed? Is it a process, or an inner sense of who we are?

Motivation Cluster

This includes achievement, drive, commitment, initiative, and optimism. [Author's Note: I would also suggest that it is about being "in mission" or principle driven. It is about being connected to something greater than ourselves, and having a sense of interconnectedness to God or a higher power.]

Vignette 10.3 describes how an educator is struggling with objectifying what is motivation and then finally figures out a way to change the approach.

Vignette 10.3

Teacher: We are going to use Cooper's (1997) EQ formula for identifying what your motivation level is for being in class today. This is called your ***motivational coefficient***. So rank yourself from 1 to 10 on how you see yourself in each of the four domains below; 1 is very low, and 10 very high. Now fill in the scores:

Calmness (C)	1–10	_____
Energy (E)	1–10	_____
Tension (T)	1–10	_____
Fatigue (F)	1–10	_____

Now calculate this formula using the numbers you presented above.

$(C \times E) - (T \times F) = M$

Your personal motivational coefficient is ***M*** = _____ .

What do you think you need to do in order to increase your motivation?

Johnny, what would you need to do to increase your motivation for being here this morning?

Johnny: I would need to go back to bed for 2 more days to reduce my fatigue, take a Xanax to ease my tension, meditate instead of coming to class to stay calm, and drink a power drink after my meditation to bring my energy back. Then I think my motivational coefficient would be in great shape.

The class breaks into laughter as many see the response by Johnny to be more insightful than the question. The teacher sees it as one of the most disappointing days he has ever had and is ruminating on his failure as a teacher as he returns to his office. He is fortunate to have a Soul Circle (Palmer, 2004) in his university, and goes to the meeting. He tells his embarrassing story. One of the members of the group, after hearing the story, asks, "Are you able to look at your intent, and how you brought the class to partner (or not) in that intent? Second, are you able to look at your hidden intent and see if it is connected to one of these three classroom approaches: (1) Student centered: What do they want?; (2) Instructor centered: What did you want?; or (3) Learning centered: What are you asking them to learn? We are here to support you in working through this challenging day in any way you need that support."

The next class with this same group: I want to let you know that during the last class, I thought there might be an easy way to look at our motivation using a formula I saw in a workshop. Johnny helped me understand that motivation in class is not as easy to address as using a formula that means different things to different people. Where the formula seems to hold up most often is in the work setting for doing a task. It has not been tested for any specific environment. The principle of *core learning* is, "What motivates students toward success in any academic activity." If that is the theme, then let's work together to see what the possible answers are for you either individually and/or collectively. Does everyone understand how this might help us learn about student motivation in classrooms even if they are different?

The key to EI and motivation is to know what motivates you, and then be willing to learn what motivates those around you. The topic of motivation is much larger than can be addressed here, but could include maturational models for readiness, psychological models, charismatic and leadership models, and behavior punishment and reward models. What triggers your motivation, and is it more objective based or subjective based? That is something worth exploring for your personal EI knowledge. Let's next consider empathy in terms of EI and SEL.

Empathy Cluster

This includes understanding others, developing others, service orientation, leveraging diversity, and political awareness. [Author's Note: I would also add that empathy is being with another in need, connection on a feeling level, and being able to feel what another is feeling without being lost in the feeling.]

The concepts of empathy are directly related to one's ability to understand what is happening to another person. Within the care paradigm, it is about being present and available. Vignette 10.4 comes from my personal life when I was learning something I had no idea existed—that the patient was teaching *me*.

Vignette 10.4

I was a senior nursing student working at the University Hospital of Wisconsin in the kidney transplant unit. Tim was my patient, and he had experienced one transplant failure and was waiting for another chance to get one more kidney. He talked, and I listened as the hair on my arms raised and my fear set in. Tim said he was sick of dialysis, a difficult process where he was hooked up to a machine three times a week for most of a day in order to filter his blood, a function the kidneys normally perform. After dialysis he would return to his room and feel sick for at least another 8 hours. His diet was totally controlled, and he couldn't have fluids because he had no kidney to take out the water. Tim was 9 years old and telling me he wanted to die. "If the next kidney fails, if there is a next kidney, I don't want to live." I sat with tears in my eyes as I do even now trying to write this story. How has he lived with so much pain in so short a time—in only 9 years? I sat and listened to a very young boy teach me about life and death. I didn't expect this. I thought I was there to help him adjust to all the medical manipulation he needed to live with this disease. No, not really! Tim became my teacher, and I went home and hugged my two daughters even more, knowing that we are not on this earth forever.

Empathy can be addressed in many ways, and going back to the workshop vignette presented earlier, it is possible to close the forgiveness exercise within this SEL domain. Vignette 10.5 demonstrates how this could play out in a faculty group.

Vignette 10.5

The group of faculty had just completed their assignment on writing a forgiveness letter as a part of the workshop. Most had written letters forgiving themselves for hanging on to what did not serve them any longer. They often spoke of removing the hook from their own flesh and giving it back to the person who gave this painful experience to them in the past. However, many were more concerned about not letting the hook stay in their flesh to fester and cause problems in other relationships.

They wrote their letters, and we walked out to the parking lot with the letter in hand, forming a circle. No one spoke, no one read the letters; it was a quiet walk. A basin sat in the center of the circle. They were asked—"Are you ready to really let go of the things you wrote down? Are you ready to burn these letters and let the universe support your personal healing? If you are, then I invite you to bring the letters forward as I start a fire in the bowl and burn them. Let the ash remind you that they have been ritually given away by you, and offer a prayer or positive thought for yourself as you let it go. You no longer need this in your life. Forgive yourself or forgive the other person who put the hook in you if possible, but burn this and let it leave you now. Let's start." Each participant came forward one at a time to burn his or her letter, many with tears in their eyes, silent, and open to being healed by their own desire for forgiving.

Let's now examine how social skills factor into SEL and education.

Social Skills Cluster

This includes influence, communication, conflict management, leadership, change catalyst, building bonds, collaboration and cooperation, and team capabilities.

The entire SEL movement is built on social skills that allow a person to deal with conflict, address difficult situations, problem solve, and collaborate to accomplish challenging tasks. Nursing is full of such challenges and there is no shortage of need. It is easy to identify a variety of times when you thought nurses failed at being socially intelligent: a nurse saying things about another nurse who is not present, giving her judgments to three other nurses on the floor; sending an email to several people about your discontent with how the administration is treating you and your unit; supporting an angry moment about the challenges of being told how to do your job differently; letting patients know you will get to them when you can because you are short staffed today.

In the classroom, an example of challenges in using social intelligence might include a teacher making an administrative announcement by saying, "This is not from me—I have to tell you this . . . ." There is no lack of social intelligence experience to draw from, but it is something quite different if we work to be more socially intelligent in what we do and that means owning our practice, owning our comments, owning our actions, and understanding that diversity is present and is a gift. Some people are not ready for certain types of information, and technology may be short-circuiting our social literacy.

What if social intelligence is deeper than we first see it—what if it includes the ability to influence, effective communication, conflict management, leadership, being a change catalyst, and building bonds and collaborating with others through team strategies (Boyatzis, Goleman, & Rhee, 1999)? Even Goleman (2006) advances the idea to include:

- *Primal empathy*: Feeling with others; sensing nonverbal emotional signals
- *Attunement*: Listening with full receptivity; attuning to a person
- *Empathic accuracy*: Understanding another person's thoughts, feelings, and intentions
- *Social cognition*: Knowing how the social world works (p. 84)

Social skills seems to be a more encompassing cluster that may even integrate all the EI clusters previously mentioned. Goleman also includes a *social facility* that involves synchrony, self-preservation, influence, and concern that suggests we be attuned to the nonverbal. It is critical to be aware of how we are presenting ourselves and influencing others, and our ability to act based on our caring about others. There is a sense of becoming competent at such skills, and again raises Hoffman's (2009) concern regarding teaching techniques and processes.

At a deeper level, a teacher may be divided from his or her self in hidden ways that are often called the *shadow self* (Goleman, 2006; Palmer, 2004; Watson, 2008). If we understood and integrated valuing our intersubjective skills, this would allow for creative discussions that are not power based or process driven (Nodding, 2006; Palmer, 2004; Watson, 2008). SEL may be a newer version of an older concept called intersubjective knowing, presented by Meed, Cooley, Blumer, and Buber (Polkinghorne, 1983). This concept describes how people connect in the moment of not knowing with no outcome of the connection. Goleman (2006) and Watson (2008) both describe this knowing in the moment of connection that was also called the *I–thou* thinking, presented by Buber, as a way to get at the intersubjective knowing that may hold one of the real truths to being socially literate. Vignette 10.6 provides an exploration of the struggle and benefits of being present for another.

Vignette 10.6

We have been studying the concepts of caring presence in this class and some ways leaders in nursing have described its application in the health care setting. The reality is, caring presence does not happen that often on most acute-care units. When nurses are asked to say why it does not normally occur, their primary response is a lack of time, too much to do, and that they just can't get it all done. Let's explore together what might be the hidden reasons that a caring presence is not common in the workplace. Some might call these the core reasons, or the archetypal needs, or just plain hidden reasons. Use your resource books, and break off into groups of four. Spend 30 minutes looking for these hidden or unconscious reasons, and write them down. Come back to the class in 30 minutes so we can explore your findings.

Now that we are all back, let's put these reasons on the board and see if we have themes from the different groups.

I want to let you know that I asked the same thing of some nurses who work at XYZ Hospital; I asked them to look at the same issues. Four of them have offered to explore what they believe are the hidden reasons they normally do not have a caring presences in their practice. We will hear them out, and then at the end ask questions from our previous discussion and findings. Keep the questions open to the possibility that they have answers we didn't get, and that they may have barriers to seeing the answers we did identify. We are all here to learn from each other because we really do not know the answers.

SUMMARY

As we have seen in this chapter, SEL is a challenging subject due to its in-depth exploration of self and the vulnerability to which a teacher is exposed by fully incorporating it into his or her teaching. However, in this chapter we have also seen the need for SEL in nursing education. It holds many attributes that are desirable in the practice of nursing and yet may be competency or process driven rather than easily integrated into who you are as a nurse. Teaching in ways that allow integration of such affective issues is not easy, and the level of integration can be identified all the way back to Krathwohl, Bloom, and Masia's (1964) taxonomy and stages of integration, which are:

1. *Receiving*: The student becomes aware and is willing to receive the affective input
2. *Responding*: The student begins acquiescence and exhibits a willingness to interact on this level
3. *Valuing*: The student accepts and expresses a preference or commitment to the topic
4. *Organization*: The student conceptualizes values and moves to an organized value system
5. *Characterization by a value complex*: The student's conceptualized value complex becomes a way of life

SEL really needs to be at stage three, four, or five to become a part of the person and their practice. To get there is certainly a role for *affective teachers* who are willing to dive into the deep unknown of their profession. However, we have guides and mentors such as Parker Palmer, Jean Watson, Daniel Goleman, Nel Nodding, and others who we would like to enlist in this journey below the surface as we explore other issues associated with affective teaching.

CHAPTER 11

International Social–Emotional Learning and the Affective Education Movement

As you might imagine, social–emotional learning (SEL) and affective education are not restricted to applications in the United States alone. These concepts have been used across the globe to varying degrees. In some cases, their application echoes what we see in the United States. In other examples, SEL can be tied to a larger political movement such as revolution and/or dealing with oppression. This chapter examines the international history of SEL and affective education and how other countries have applied them in the classroom. There is some confusion in language and the background agenda for many of the international educational reform movements, but the ones presented here can be defined as SEL and/or affective education throughout the world. Some of the larger global themes encompass Europe, Chile, and the Asian Pacific rim. Lang (1998) puts the European views of affective education into context on several levels. First, he believes the student and the teacher are humans with emotions and feelings that need some care and respect in order to achieve their best educational outcomes. In addition, he believes there is a need to go beyond the traditional academic model in order to nurture an autonomous student that will contribute to the overall societal needs and live a fulfilled life. Lang finds the natural integration of affective classroom strategies as having social–emotional learning (SEL) attributes.

> It is impossible to teach without the courage to love, without the courage to try a thousand times before giving in. In short, it is impossible to teach without a forged, invented, and well-thought-out capacity to love. (Freire, 1998)

He states: "The objective of the personal and social dimension of the curriculum includes enabling pupils to:

- Learn to respect and value themselves and others
- Appreciate the benefits of resolving conflict by nonviolent means
- Learn to tell the difference between intention and action
- Learn to tolerate and the need to take responsibility for their own behavior" (p. 10)

This example shows the integration of SEL and affective teaching in the European community during the mid- to late-1990s. As early as 1970, Paulo Freire wrote about the problems seen in the Chilean educational system and wrote a classic book titled *Pedagogy of the Oppressed.* This was a time of social revolution and academic revolt. Freire (1970/2009) states, "Education as the exercise of domination stimulates the credulity of students, with the ideological intent (often not perceived by educators) of indoctrinating them to adapt to the world of oppression" (p. 78). He describes this form of teaching as the *banking model,* which is reactionary, and emphasizes permanence instead of change. Freire was one of the first to espouse *learning-centered* classrooms that used real social problems as case studies to solve, and then had the students conduct reflective personal values clarification on themselves. This process was called "dialogical teaching" (p. 17), where each classroom experience was converted to a dialogue involving what was learned, possible theoretical outcomes learned, and what the students learned regarding themselves. Not only was Freire an international educational leader, but he offered exceptional methods that would easily be defined as affective pedagogical methods.

The Asia and the Pacific Programme of Educational Innovation for Development (APEID, 1992) examined the need for affective educational development and looked at what was already in place at the time with an emphasis on children and youth in the Asia and Pacific regions. Their intent was to explore affective education, which was seen as:

> . . . a domain of education where feelings and attitudes come to play. However, it is a domain not very well understood . . . yet its importance has been stressed in the world's great religions and emphasized, time and time again, by great philosophers and teachers. (p. i)

This affective education and research continued from these early periods through the current day, and therefore we have seen fluctuations with increases and decreases of activity occurring when speaking of international SEL and affective education. In addition, there may be many holes in this international view, as only English documents or those translated into English were used for references in this text. However, as we will see in this chapter, an examination of how social–emotional intelligence and affective education are treated internationally, which gives us a broader perspective on applying these concepts in the classroom. In many cases, affective education has been implemented across the globe for political and social reasons. And, as with their implementation in the United States, effective strategies for implementing SEL and affective education can be challenging. (Dr. Maurice Elias presents the need for SEL in this video clip, www.youtube.com/watch?v=7K2uSg-_KlI&feature=youtu.be.)

AFFECTIVE EDUCATION IN ASIA AND THE PACIFIC REGIONS

There are two areas that will be covered here as a way to provide the reader with an overview of affective education in the Asia and Pacific region: history and research. The more historical section comes from the APEID (1992), which gives an overview of China, Indonesia, Malaysia, Nepal, the Philippines, Sri Lanka, and Thailand. Unfortunately there are few references on SEL or affective education for this region. It would also be valuable to have an update on how Indochina is doing today, but such documents could not be found at the time of this writing. In addition, the historical documentation addresses primarily children and youth education versus higher education, but it will give some perspective on what the issues are in various countries. The second area is what type of research addressing the affective domain related to higher education is currently being conducted in the particular region of the world.

China

China's affective teaching methods are primarily absent, as this is a culture that has had its focus on cognitive learning domains with instructional methods, which have been called *duck-feeding* and *preaching* (APEID, 1992). The affective teaching interventions that were to be implemented focused on moral education programs and regulated the behaviors of primary school teachers to model social problem resolutions and the use of field visits to learn by watching real-world issues.

Indonesia

Indonesia has a constitutional statement from 1945 that provides universal education for all young people and citizens. It was based on tenets similar to the United States' early doctrine that was God focused and addressed the attributes of a good citizen, which included supporting the national spirit and love of country. There was a 1970 reform of the educational system by the Indonesian Ministry of Education and Culture that aimed at improving the quality of education and provided the guidelines for what a good teacher must be. In addition, the Ministry saw education as having the historical three domains of affective, cognitive, and psychomotor.

By 1980, additional changes for improved education were instituted, which were called the Active Learning and Professional Support (ALPS) project. This process changed classrooms by focusing on more critical thinking activities, use of proxemics for stimulating learning environments, seeing the students as unique and different, and using the classroom environment as a learning tool. Teachers were given special training and had formal education plans. The teachers also had clubs and learning centers for themselves. The third domain of ALPS was to encourage the community to better understand the importance of education for their young people. It suggested there were many ways in which the community could be involved to support the overall learning process of children. Indonesia had a specific agenda for supporting the affective domain of learning and used these strategies in the late 1980s.

Malaysia

Malaysia became an independent state in 1957 and its educational goals stemmed from the need for national unity that was reinforced by the formation of the Rukunegara (the national philosophy) in 1970. The national unity priority gave a strong message to young people about what it means to be supporters of the belief in God and loyalty to the king. However, in 1983, the national syllabus, called the Civics Syllabus, was replaced by the Moral Education Syllabus in order to give students a better education in values development. The Moral Education Syllabus took the traditional 3Rs emphasis and added intellectual problem solving and sensitivity awareness to the aesthetics in the environment and the emotions of self and others. The approach incorporated both direct and indirect SEL teaching methods. The instructional methods used were:

- Problem-solving techniques
- Use of models and paradigms
- Simulation games
- Drama
- Discussion
- Case studies
- Project work, and so forth (APEID, 1992, p. viii)

Teachers were trained in the use of affective pedagogy for student development that integrated traditional academic knowledge and SEL issues.

Nepal

In Nepal, the primary role of the educator is to teach the young person in cognitive development and to shape the personality of the child. There is no expressed push to teach SEL or to use affective teaching methods. However, there are significant moral educational lessons that may be seen as being focused on affective personality development. So, in Nepal, whatever happens in the affective domain is an accidental result of the need to address the moral development of the child.

Philippines

In contrast to what we see in Nepal, the Philippines has been concerned with affective education since the early 1900s. They use different language for SEL skills and development called character building activities (CBA) and rules of urbanity that are tied to moral ways of being with self and others. This includes such domains as self-actualization, being in community, being productive in society, national commitment and pride, and faith in God. There was one affective development model rolled out to most of the country, which was used to promote a positive attitude toward work, a vocation, and a sense of valuing a productive life and nation. They implemented this with some unique service-learning curricular changes that moved learning to the neighborhoods.

Teacher education in the Philippines has also been extensive to incorporate understanding and use of the curriculum-based assessment (CBA) model and to include parents in this teaching model. They also have used group dynamics for students as a way to process and learn from each other. As a result, Filipinos actively link affective and cognitive educational methods and content as a natural part of their educational system.

Thailand

There seems to be a disconnect in Thailand between the desire to have affective teaching and actually having it. It has been overshadowed by significant cognitive achievement and expectations by parents in this culture. There is an expectation to integrate 30 moral characters into the lives of each child, but much of this is expected to come from the parents and not the schools. They would also argue that affective development is an ongoing process and it is not likely to see a special academic strategy for integration into its young people.

Higher Education in China

In China, a pivotal and unique research study by Shen, Wang, and Shen (2009) was performed. These researchers examined the use of emotional data to increase e-learning. This study involved online college students who were set up to provide a biophysical signal back to the instructor that could tell what state of emotion the student was in as lessons progressed. The most common states were engagement and confusion, but the key is that these emotions were easily seen by the instructor to guide student learning. This study found that when the instructor could adapt to the emotional state of the student, it did have a significant impact on learning. These authors also address two critical issues for online education. First, there is a significant loss for the instructor who may be using facial expressions and body language to guide students, and second, if there is a way to get emotional feedback to an instructor working online, the instructor can still make adjustments to increase the learning of the student.

This shows an interesting blend between the current issues of e-learning and the value of having affective teaching methods integrated into such learning. There are certainly other issues to address with respect to the integration of affective pedagogy for e-learning, which was presented in Chapter 7.

AFFECTIVE EDUCATION IN EUROPE

There is little documentation for affective teaching in Europe; the primary resource is information that was collected by Lang, Katz, and Menezes (1998). The work of Lang et al. (1998) presents many expert opinions from a host of countries by senior education leaders from their area of the world. Some language and concepts are very difficult to translate into Western educational thinking, and that discussion will not be delved into, but one example of a European educational concept will be pointed out, as it relates to SEL. *Wychowanie* in Polish literature means "purposeful activity of some people aiming to cause permanent changes in the other people's personalities through interaction" (Muszynski, 1977 in Lang, Katz, & Menezes, p. 11). *Wychowanie* is an interesting way to phrase how one might attempt to impact the personality development of another person, or to even have a responsibility to do so through affective education. This is an obvious risk for how one might use affective teaching methods to control a population, and do so with long-lasting results.

Lang (1998) states, "The term 'affective education' is adopted not because of its conceptual power, but because it is the term that made some sense to all the European countries involved in the collaborative work of which this book is one outcome" (p. 12). In addition to creating an understanding of affective education, Lang also clarifies that he uses a three-level model to create additional understanding of what countries are doing. The levels are:

1. Reaction/cure: "Doing something after the problem has arisen . . ." (p. 13)
2. Proaction/prevention: "Doing something before the event by preparing people to cope with anticipated situations . . ." (p. 13)
3. Enhancement: "Positive encouragement of development, not primarily driven by the desirability of prevention, but by the aim of developing the whole person . . ." (p. 13).

The first two levels do not match with previously stated definitions of affective education. However, in keeping with the goals of this text, one can look at which countries are accomplishing affective education within the *enhancement* level as described by Lang. The descriptions that follow examine accomplishments in Lang's third level regarding enhancement.

Germany

Much of the German educational system looks at the powerful influence of the relationship between the student and the teacher. In addition, Dreesmann (1982) focused on the classroom environment and stressed the need to explore the ability to measure affective and subjective realities within the classroom. His conclusion was, "The personal relations between the pupils in the class and their teacher as well as pupil interrelations are of great importance for pupils while the teaching subject and its instruction play a secondary role" (p. 98). Similarly, Fess (1998) states, "There can be no doubt therefore that affective objectives are of significance, not only for the well-being of the pupils, but for their academic performance as well" (p. 31). German educators have based their educational foundation on two major themes. The first is that each child is an independent learner and can learn by being exposed to a variety of experiences and knowledge. The second theme is the idea that each child is a holistic being that is more than a vessel to fill with knowledge or facts. Both themes support the idea of social learning and primarily focus on the K–10 grades. These constructs have been the support for *child-centered* and *holistic* pedagogy using teaching methods such as team or small-group learner models that started with Germany's Koln–Holweide and Gottingen–Geismar programs as early as 1976.

Contrary to what we find regarding social learning in K–10 education in Germany, there is minimal information as to the impact of this social learning on higher education or the students in higher education settings. Vocational and technical schools had a primary focus on skill development for a career and do not have any expectation of creating a relational learning environment. Thus, although there is a great deal of emphasis on social learning for younger students, the entire affective process seems to end with secondary education in Germany.

Ireland

The school system in Ireland is broken down into first level or K–8 grades, second level or secondary school, and third level or higher education. In 1996, there was an official launching of the Irish Association of Pastoral Care in Education (IAPCE) arising out of an official gathering of educators in 1994 at Dublin Castle. Pastoral care was the term given for affective education. Not only was affective education seen as important, but there was a structure put in place that allowed for affective education to be in the schools (Collins, 1998).

Some of the courses found within the context of pastoral care education involved counseling skills for teachers and in-service days for the entire staff to focus on this topic. The pastoral care courses were aimed at personal and social development. Prior to these more recent events, Ireland was primarily the recipient of Catholic indoctrination and 800 years of Irish/English history that was filled with various levels of positive and negative political events that kept hampering the building of a consistent educational model.

England

Starting in the late 18th century, there has been a desire on the part of British educators to be child focused and to educate the *whole child*. However, the struggle for educators on England rests on the practical tradition of being focused on subject knowledge dissemination and maintaining discipline, versus their more recent desire to address the affective domain of the student as one might expect when dealing with the whole child. Best (1998) describes this confusing struggle between a desire to integrate Krathwohl et al.'s (1964) definition of affective teaching outcomes and the formal presence and authoritarian classrooms found in England from the 1950s to the late 1990s. All the words, strategies, and desires were in place, but it was difficult to see real changes in their educational strategies.

Some affective influences came from the training of educators to the humanistic therapy approaches presented by Rogers (1961), which allowed many British educators to integrate this approach into the classroom. This allowed the schools to have resident counselors available for all students, and some of these strategies made it into the curriculum. However, affective teaching methods were fragmented and inconsistent and gradually were removed in the 1970s and 1980s. So many innovative practices started and stopped, including the Humanities Curriculum Project, Pastoral Carers programs, Active Tutorial Work, and more (Best, 1998). In some cases, affective education was introduced through traditional classes, which was often a natural and accepted way of teaching some courses. This included:

- The development of aesthetic appreciation through art, music, and literature
- The promotion of empathy through literature and history, and the accompanying development of moral concepts and dispositions
- The development, appreciation, expression, and control of the emotions through educational drama
- The mastery of such emotions and dispositions as timidity and the fear of physical intimidation through games and physical education
- Opportunities to reflect upon more or less deeply felt feelings of spirituality and religious belief in religious education
- Growing self-confidence and self-understanding achieved through any subject where the pedagogy is appropriate (p. 78)

When examining these strategies, these educators in England were at the forefront of affective teaching methods for this period and were doing so without really formally addressing these strategies as affective pedagogy. Another significant issue is that there is no mention of such education in postsecondary schools, even as an unstated by-product of conventional teaching. Best ends his discussion with, "There is, I think, a relative neglect of the emotions in the mainstream of U.K. schooling" (p. 80) and he believes it may be related to the traditions arising out of the Enlightenment in European culture.

Russia

Russia has a confusing history with affective education, and it continues to be confusing today. The early efforts were tied to the humanizing psychology that actually started in the 18th century with Peter the Great, but that was abandoned after Peter the Great's reign and was all but completely absent until 1954. From 1954 to 1958, psychology was placed back in the curriculum of many schools in Russia, but in 1958 it was no longer mandatory and became an area only examined and researched by psychologists. Russia has been through significant societal changes in the past 30 years, causing a significant hampering of educational research activities. This has led to minimal movement of strategies for using affective teaching within any part of the Russian academic system (Zabrodin, Popova, & Minaev, 1998).

Spain

Spain's educational system can be viewed as having two distinct periods with the first being during the dictatorship of Franco prior to 1975. In 1970 with the introduction of the Villas Law, the education system was reformed to provide free basic education that included education in private schools. However, it was not until the country was in democratic reform starting in 1975 with a new constitution in 1978, that sweeping reforms occurred, which included the freedom of conscious approach and the participation of teachers, parents, and students in the pursuit of religious and moral education that was value-based. In short, the constitutional changes moved education into a democratic process that included fundamental rights often seen in democratic societies (Ballesteros, 1989). The educational reforms were directly tied to the societal changes within Spain and the General Ordination Law of the Educational System, called LOGSE 1990, which promoted three domains that were tied to the affective development of the students:

- To awake in the pupil the joy of living
- To promote attitudes that encourage the development of individuals who can live in harmony with themselves and with others
- To create a homogeneous society in which social relationships are more harmonious and greater humanity exists (Pampliega & Marroquin, 1998, p. 85)

SUMMARY

Affective educational strategies in other parts of the world all seem to be tied to the political climate and social development of those countries. In any one area, there may have been variations over time that supported the use of affective pedagogy in the form of cultural moral development. In several cases, it was tied to the use of psychology as a basic tenet of education, and then disappeared in parallel with psychology in the curriculum. Very little is offered in the way of pedagogy for faculty to use in the classrooms.

What this chapter does point to is an international belief in SEL and affective education that struggles for a rightful place in current education across the world. It has offered some important values for educators and governments on what is effective and good teaching, but lacks a philosophy that has deeply become foundational to the world's view of education. This continues to represent the struggle for SEL and affective teaching methods through world history, including that of the United States, and how difficult it is to maintain this domain of educational pedagogy.

CHAPTER 12

Taking the Red Pill and Breaking the Illusions

A new type of teacher is one that is connected authentically to his or her soul and has the ability to be present in the classroom. I call this the *soulful teacher.* A *soulful teacher* is concerned for the soul of his or her students as described by Glazer (1999), Moore (1940, reproduced in 1992), and Watson (2008). Moore believes the care of the soul is found in the way we love, form attachments, and how we build and form relationships. Based on recent studies in caring already discussed, the care of the soul would also show up in our ability to *care* in the broadest sense, meaning that you bring your authentic self into the classroom (Koerner, 2007; Nodding, 2005; Watson, 2008). Teachers who are *caring* in the classroom would be defined as *soulful teachers,* as they do their inner work, understand their hidden selves, strive to be openly authentic, allow for intersubjective learning, and are able to lessen fear of decision making in their practices. There is a deep and perhaps unconscious volcano hidden below the surface that has kept many teachers from being in connection to his or her soul work of teaching. To expose this hidden paralysis means we have to take a risk.

> When the soul is neglected, it doesn't just go away; it appears symptomatically in obsessions, addictions, violence, and loss of meaning. . . . Fulfilling work, rewarding relationships, personal power, and relief from symptoms are all gifts of the soul. (Moore, 1940/1992, p. xi)

THE RED PILL OR THE BLUE PILL

This is the time to sit, reflect, and make a choice, as Neo did in the movie *The Matrix* when he was asked by Morpheus, did he want to stay in the illusion of what he thought was real, or did he want to be forever changed? If he took the blue pill, all would stay the same, and he could wake up tomorrow and believe everything was just as he thought it always had been. If he took the red pill, the world would never be seen the same way again. A clip regarding this critical moment for Neo from the movie *The Matrix* is at http://www.youtube.com/watch?v=zE7PKRjrid4&feature=youtu.be.

You too have a choice about the future of your teaching. You could have stopped reading this text long before this point. Maybe you had to read this for a course and you are now ready to sell the book and move on to another course. You can take the blue pill and have some good ideas as to what you might do in your future as a teacher and you will wake up tomorrow thinking in the same way you did prior to starting this journey of the authentic and soulful teacher. So, what has brought you to this point? Have you already been nibbling on the red pill? If so, you might as well swallow it and break all the illusions related to what keeps your teaching as it is, or what it would take to change it—some subconscious soul work.

A NEW PROFESSIONAL

If you are considering the red pill, do not do this alone. Find a support group in your teaching environment where more of your colleagues are also taking the red pill and are ready to break the illusions of what they believe is real. Maybe it is a *learning community* (Samaras, Freese, Kosnik, & Beck, 2008), a *Caritas learning community* (Watson, 2008), or a *circle of trust* (Palmer, 2004). Each of these types of support groups offers a safe place to share and receive ideas and critiques of your teaching. As we will see later in our discussion regarding the shadow self, such a safety net is essential when we take the red pill and begin to develop our healthy authentic selves. Together, you will find not only help and safe support for the journey but also a motivation to keep going. Such motivation is key to truly transforming our teaching.

> Most will continue to lie low because they fear reprisals or are so overworked that they lack time and energy for advocacy. A vigilant public that speaks truth to power will always be needed. (Palmer, 2007, p. 203)

In keeping with the theme of transformation, it is time to start the *new profession* that is presented by Palmer (2007). "Most will continue to lie low because they fear reprisals or are so overworked that they lack time and energy for advocacy. A vigilant public that speaks truth to power will always be needed" (p. 203). Palmer suggests that this new approach to teaching will require a new profession with five goals:

1. We must help our students debunk the myth that institutions possess autonomous, even ultimate, power over our lives.
2. We must validate the importance of our students' emotions as well as their intellect. (creates affective literacy)
3. We must teach our students how to "mine" their emotions for knowledge. (increases affective literacy)
4. We must teach the students how to cultivate community for the sake of both knowing and doing.
5. We must teach—and model for our students—what it means to be on the journey toward "an undivided life." (p. 205)

DEEPENING THE JOURNEY

I intend to speak boldly about what might be the real reason educators have not addressed affective literacy in their students. Why do we teach in traditional *teacher-centered* ways, even when we know it is poor teaching? What is it about my inner self that says I cannot change my teaching? Why hasn't the academy pushed for faculty to change from the teacher-centered model after all these years, or why do we believe technology is our answer? Moore (1940/1992) suggests that we as teachers are disconnected from our souls. Most teachers are the antithesis of *soulful teachers.* Moore says it this way:

> It is commonplace for writers to point out that we live in a time of deep division, in which mind is separate from body, and that spirituality is at odds with materialism. . . . We cannot just think ourselves through it, because thinking itself is part of the problem. (p. xiii)

Palmer (2007) continues with telling his readers that this quest is not one where we find a "path away from the shadow of death."

> A soulful personality is complicated, multifaceted and shaped by both pain and pleasure, success and failure. Life lived soulfully is not without its moments of darkness and periods of foolishness. Dropping the salvational fantasy frees us up to the possibility of self-knowledge and self-acceptance, which are the very foundations of soul. (pp. xvi, xvii)

Watson (2008) states that nurses are a work in progress, but as we approach *Caritas literacy* we will develop the following:

- Cultivate caring consciousness and intentionality as a starting point
- Ability to "center"—quiet down, pause before entering a patient's room or be still in the presence of the other
- Ability to "read the field" when entering into the life space or field of another

- Ability to be present—be with the other as well as do for others
- Accurately identify and address persons by name
- Maintain eye contact as appropriate for person/cultural meaning and sensitivity
- Ability to ground self and others for comforting, soothing, calming acts
- Accurately detect the feelings of others
- Stay within the other's frame of reference
- Invite and authentically listen to the inner meaning—the subjective story of others
- Hold the other with an attitude of unconditional loving—kindness, equanimity, dignity, and regard
- Ability to be with "silence," waiting for the other to reflect before responding to questions, allowing the other's inner thoughts to emerge
- Respond to the other's feelings and mood verbally and nonverbally, with authentic affective congruence (p. 25)

Look at the emotional and social intelligence Watson is asking nurses to strive for. In addition, she is asking for nurses to show up in the healthy authentic self for the other—our patients, our students, our families.

If we are able to see where the soul is connecting and present by the behaviors presented earlier, then it is also possible to see the symptoms within a classroom when it is absent. The classroom cannot be pain free, and most would argue that it should never be. The place of pain is often a clinical sign of where to be more observant. If we are speaking of a student, then it would be a good thing that the student observes where and how he or she is learning, growing, or changing—all of which might cause some pain. If we are speaking of an instructor having pain, then this too is a place of learning, growth, or change occurring within the instructor. What a great sense of awareness for a teacher who is in alignment with his or her soul to sense some painful growth. The authentic teacher takes a risk in this approach, and as Weimer (2010) states, "Conduct in and out of the classroom conveys messages about values, beliefs, and attitudes, about teachers as human beings. These personal expressions make teachers vulnerable and teaching risky" (p. 9). We must continue to explore why teachers would take the risk and what it really means to care for one's students.

In order to better understand the risks we undertake in caring for our students, it is worthwhile to examine the types of care that we can have in the classroom. There are two forms of care that originated with Heidegger's philosophy of care (Heidegger, 1962). The first is a process where you care enough and are skilled enough to take over for someone who is incapable of doing so for him or herself. This could occur in a clinical sense with an unconscious patient, or in a classroom where the student does not know the path to knowledge in a particular area.

The second level of care is the ability to pull back and let the patient or student do self-care or self-learning, and the person caring gives back the responsibility and mentored skill to the client or student. Nursing students are taught how to care for those who are unable to care for themselves, and they are taught how to address self-care deficit knowledge through patient teaching. What can cause a risk to both types of caring is the teacher/clinician's need for power and self-preservation because of fragile inner psychic awareness—a wounded soul in the teacher. When this occurs, many things fall apart as described by Halldorsdottir (1990) in her chapter called "The Essential Structure of a Caring and an Uncaring Encounter With a Teacher: The Perspective of the Nursing Student."

Many of us who are now nursing educators may have had experiences that can be described from both perspectives—the caring and the uncaring, as presented by Halldorsdottir. She describes the caring teacher as "professionally competent, has genuine concern for the student as a studying person, has a positive personality, and is professionally committed" (p. 97). Such teachers build mutual trust and formulate relationships between them and the students, which encompass a *respectful distance*. These attributes are very similar to immediacy theory practices for effective teaching found in the field of communications. In either case, the teacher is being asked to step up to his or her authentic caring self in order to establish a relationship with the student that will have many positive learning outcomes.

The fear-driven teacher shows up and creates the opposite student responses. Fear may be related to feelings of incompetence, lack of personal concern for others because the self is in crisis, the need to control or exert power in order to feel safe, or a type of initiation to a perceived rite-of-passage the teacher believes the student must go through. Singham (2007) states:

> The typical syllabus gives little indication that the students and teacher are embarking on an exciting learning adventure together, and its tone is more akin to something that might be handed to a prisoner on the first day of incarceration. (p. 52)

All of these uncaring teaching approaches create negative outcomes on the part of the student. The challenge in shifting this teaching approach occurs because it creates a divided self for that instructor. The problem is that this divided self is full of fear, self-doubt, need for additional safety, and uncaring teaching behaviors, which may be flowing from the shadow side of self—the hidden, unconscious self (Hall & Nordby, 1973; Palmer, 2007). *The work must begin with the teacher individually and what has brought him or her to this career using the methods you do.* The authentic self by itself is not acceptable for *soulful teachers* even though it is necessary. We do not want the Mr. Hyde showing up in the classroom.

We want Dr. Jekyll to be there. A movie trailer from the story is found at http://www.youtube.com/watch?v=wbg5oXpq42Y. This clip highlights the idea that good and evil both lurk within us. Thinking that we all may have a dark side is not easy for some to understand, but others know this to be true. However, Parker (1999) also suggests that both are part of the same person, but one is the dark shadow side that is not conscious. "The second thing I didn't learn [in school]—and this takes me even more deeply inward—is that there is within me, in the shadow of my own soul, a little Hitler, a force of evil" (pp. 25–26). Nodding (2005) warns the teacher of the same thing by stating:

> We live in an age both blessed and encumbered by a new orthodoxy in speech. . . . We are properly aware that words can hurt badly and even inflict real and lasting harm. But as our language is purged, our fears, misgivings, and dislikes sink into a layer of the psyche that Carl Jung (1933) called the *shadow*. This is the individual and collective side we deny. Continuous denial does not destroy the shadow. It stays with us, and sometimes creates spontaneous explosions of verbal and physical violence. (p. 120)

The same is true for students who are in need of faculty who understand the complex issues in today's vulnerable world where students may also be showing their shadow side. Kirman (1977) stated, "Only by attending to the individual unconscious needs of students, can we hope to reach out to that vast majority of children and young adults for whom school is still a less that meaningful passing of time" (p. v). Kirman also believes educators need this shadow awareness because he states, "Of course, an individual cannot be truly loving until he has the capacity to be truly hating in a controlled way" (p. 5). It would appear that we need this level of awareness to finally be conscious and authentic and, at the same time, creating a place of choice.

[*This is a good time to drink more water to wash down the red pill even farther*].

As we start to own our shadow side, we can take the shadow out of hiding—own it—and ask this part of us to have a better purpose in our lives. This means I can know how I can hate, but now I have a conscious choice to love even more deeply instead of hate. It does not mean that I will be more likely to hate, but rather, when I feel hate come over me, I can choose to face it differently. I can love even more.

Here are some psychoanalytic explanations of what is meant by "shadow."

Many writers (Jung in Hall & Nordby, 1973; Bly, 1988; Jacobi, 1973; Zweig & Abrams, 1991) dealing with the issue of shadow, place it into the psychoanalytical framework of unconscious where it is often projected onto others. It can be seen as positive and negative attributes of self, but is simply that part of our unconscious that we cannot accept and therefore we put it on others. Zweig and Abrams have collected writings from over 40 authors who have written on some aspects of the shadow in their text called *Meeting the Shadow: The Hidden Power of the Dark Side of Human Nature*. Hillman, who is a Jungian analyst and currently writes on the issues of the shadow, is quoted as saying, "The unconscious cannot be conscious; the moon has its dark side, the sun goes down and cannot shine everywhere at once, and even God has two hands. Attention and focus require some things to be out of the field of vision, to remain in the dark. One cannot look both ways" (Zweig & Abrams, 1991, pp. XVII–XVIII). Zweig and Abrams describe the integration of the shadow as *shadow-work*. "Shadow-work is the conscious and intentional process of admitting to that which we have chosen to ignore or repress" (p. 239).

The shadow side of self causes the competent and caring educator to have a dark side that keeps showing up if that part of self has never been integrated properly. Teachers who are unable to integrate the suppressed self, the unconscious self, or the hidden self run the risk of seriously acting out experiences that are very destructive to self or those around them. This means we want the *conscious authentic* self to show up in *soulful teachers*. This would be described as a teacher who has integrated enough of his or her own unconscious self in a way that the teacher can be present for others in an authentic caring way. Fear will slowly be removed and caring behaviors will be present more often as the dark energy is given a new role in the life of the teacher. This energy transfer could be called *scripting a new life* for this dark energy once the teacher knows what it looks like. The key is to do enough of your own personal work so these attributes show up in a healthy authentic way—as a natural reflection of who you are, where the darker side can be safely released in a special *learning community*, a *Caritas learning community*, or a *circle of trust*. You will notice if you have the shadow in balance once you are showing immediacy, care, or caritas practices in the classroom. Affective pedagogy allows the instructor to bring these attributes to the classroom in a smooth and seamless manner. These actions cannot be forced or they will be noticed as such and will be rejected because they are inauthentic.

Consider the power of the support group safety net in creating authentic practices in the classroom through the new member's journey presented in Vignette 12.1.

Vignette 12.1

Teacher Support Group: Meeting every other week for 2 hours.

We have a new member joining today. As you know, the requirements are to read a book on shadow, and then bring a teacher reflection to this group to discuss "one-step-back" and then have the person attempt to look at his or her "two-step-back" process as best as possible while in the group.

As a reminder, nothing at this meeting can be repeated outside of these meetings, and you are only allowed to discuss your own self-awareness experiences outside this room. Let's repeat our mission and purpose for this meeting: "We are here, knowing we are all connected. We are able to become aware of what was hidden to us, and having this awareness supports the conscious authentic teacher within us."

Welcome! Tell us about your journey to this gathering of care teachers.

I have had students know me so well, they were open to giving me honest feedback by saying, "You look really stressed today. Are you okay?" It was obvious I did not prepare my inner self for that class because my emotional energy was all over my face and body—I brought the wrong teacher to the classroom. I thanked the students for letting me know this so that I could readjust and calibrate this energy that was still attached to me. I find it amazing, humbling, and a benefit if I have students who can tell me my pant zipper is down at the beginning of a class and not hint to it at break 50 minutes later, or tell me my negative energy is sitting on my face and maybe I want to do something about that before class starts. I see such openness between students and instructor as creating an authentic classroom where I also get to learn what I may unconsciously be bringing to this learning environment.

When the students raise the authenticity bar in the classroom, the instructor has at least two choices: (1) go into an ineffective coping state such as denial, projection, or hiding, or (2) step up to the reality that each person is learning and that faculty also have knowledge deficits and embarrassing experiences that can also produce learning moments for them. My hope would be that every teacher can always say, "Well, what can I learn from that experience?" Here is a chance to practice the second choice using this Vignette 12.2.

Vignette 12.2

You are caught wearing one black and one dark blue shoe that are identical in shape. A student says, "Your shoes are different colors." You say. . . . (What comes to mind? Write it here.)

Try this response:

"Thanks for telling me. I appreciate your helping me where I might not be awake. I need to remember this about myself during class today as well. It may show up in other ways, so thanks again."

As students open up to an authentic and open classroom, anything can happen so get ready and stop taking it personally. Another example is seen in Vignette 12.3.

Vignette 12.3

You have a blouse button that is not buttoned. A student says, "You have a button that is not fastened." Think to yourself "Well, what can I learn from this experience?" You might say to the student, "I was hoping to only discuss self-disclosure today, and not demonstrate it. Thanks for telling me this. I might need to keep a closer eye on my topic today than I anticipated."

Be open to the possibility for student feedback being immediately provided to you in the classroom because it could be coming. If you have never had such open feedback in a classroom, it could be a little shocking. I also believe many faculty may fear such openness in the classroom for the very reasons I have just described—it creates highly open and direct feedback for the instructor in the moment.

> I deny my inner darkness, giving it more power over me, or I project it onto other people, creating "enemies" where none exist. (Palmer, 2004, pp. 4–5)

Palmer (1999) believes the best way to bring the teacher back to the sacredness of teaching and the teaching relationship is to:

- Be aware that each of us has come from our own type of dark society and cultural biases, which means we need to learn how this impacts our beliefs and behaviors
- Be aware of our own internal little Hitler, and that we have a shadow and dark side that can easily be let out
- Be aware that when we recover the sacred, we recover our sense of community and this is the heart of good teaching
- Be aware that when we recover the sacred, we recover the humility that makes teaching and learning possible
- Be aware that when we recover the sacred, we recover our capacity for wonder and surprise (Palmer, in Glazer pp. 25–29)

Palmer defines the sacred as "that which is worthy of respect" (p. 20). He believes we can practice this at any time and in the moment once we understand it. Unfortunately, Palmer sees academia plagued by fear as the primary motivator for teachers. If each teacher is able to take on his or her need for reclaiming the sacred in all things, each will become passionate regarding building connections and relationships that will be respectful and humbled by the differences we have as we seek learning-centered classrooms. In addition, we need to reflect back on what it means to have classrooms that promote affective literacy for the students. The definition we used earlier in this text suggests that affective pedagogy requires that educators become much more aware of what is going on inside of them during their teaching moments. This definition, found in Chapter 1, is the individual's integration of knowledge regarding emotion, preference, choice, feeling, belief, attitude, ethics, and personal awareness of the self.

The current topic could not be more relevant to meet the affective literacy of the instructors who wish to be *soulful teachers*. To have such inner awareness is extraordinary, risky, difficult, and even painful for teachers on this journey.

The academy does not typically have environments encompassing safe places for educators to gather together and flush out unconscious behaviors that are affecting faculty, where there are no significant power differentials or where there are safe ways to challenge one's assumptions using critical reflection. However, we are seeing a less aggressive movement where issues are not as deep but other versions of faculty support are provided through a *learning community*, a *Caritas learning community*, or a *circle of trust*.

We fear affective education methods for many possible reasons and the biggest risk is that affective teaching sounds like educational therapy—and maybe it is. How can faculty take such risks in their classrooms? How would they address the criticism of bringing psychotherapy to their classes? How will we create an academy that will value faculty growth in the affective domain as well as student development toward affective literacy? Well, it is too late for you—you have already taken the red pill, so you will either take some safe actions toward being a *soulful teacher* as you create care pedagogy for your students, or you might take larger steps. I recommend doing the larger steps in some locations where there is personal support for *the red pill explorers* like yourself.

Epilogue

Thanks to all of you who have taken this journey with me to the land of *soulful teachers, affective teachers,* and *learning-centered classrooms.* It is hoped that everyone received some gifts and tools from this book that will serve each of you in your own way and at any level you wish. Welcome to all of you who are passionate about increasing affective literacy, about putting the authentic soul into our teaching, and who are on this journey as *soulful teachers.* Thanks for joining me. Thanks for taking the red pill.

References

American Association of Colleges of Nursing (2009, February 19). *Nurse faculty tool kit for the implementation of the baccalaureate essentials.* At http://www.aacn.nche.edu/Education/pdf/BacEssToolkit.pdf. Retrieved on 6/4/11.

Ariely, D. (2012). *The honest truth about dishonesty: How we lie to everyone—especially ourselves.* New York, NY: HarperCollins Publishing.

Arntz, W., Chasse, B., & Vicente, M. (2005). *What the bleep do you know? Discovering the endless possibilities for altering your everyday reality.* Deerfield Beach, FL: Health Communications, Inc.

Asia and the Pacific Programme of Educational Innovation for Development (APEID). (1992). Education for affective development: A guidebook on programmes and practices. Bangkok: UNESCO Principal Regional Office for Asia and the Pacific.

Ballesteros, R. (1989). Introduction: La educacion tras la recuperacion de la demoracia en Espana: 1978–1988. In P. Lang, Y. Katz, & I. Menezes (Eds.), Affective education: A comparative view (pp. 85–98). London: Cassell. Barchard, K. (2003, October). Does emotional intelligence assist in the prediction of academic success? *Educational and Psychological Measurement, 63*, 840–858.

Barone, T. E. (1992). On the demise of subjectivity in educational inquiry. *Curriculum Inquiry, 22*, pp. 25–38.

Barr, R. B. (1998, September/October). Obstacles in implementing the learning paradigm: What it takes to overcome them. *About Campus, 3*(4), 18–25.

Beane, J. A. (1990). *Affect in the curriculum: Toward democracy, dignity, and diversity.* New York, NY: Teachers College Press.

Beisser, A. (1970). The paradoxical theory of change. In J. Fagan & I. Shepherd (Eds.), *Gestalt therapy now* (pp. 77–88). New York, NY: Harper and Row.

Benner, P., Sutphen, M., Leonard, V., & Day, L. (2010). *Educating nurses: A call for radical transformation.* San Francisco, CA: Jossey-Bass.

Bernard, R. M., Abrami, P. C., Borokhovski, E., Wade, C. A., Tamim, R. M., Surkes, M. A., & Bethel, E. C. (2009, September). A meta-analysis of three types of interaction treatments in distance education. *Review of Educational Research, 79*(3), 1243–1289.

Bertrand, Y. (2003). *Contemporary theories and practice in education* (2nd ed.). Madison, WI: Atwood Publishing.

Best, R. (1998). The development of affective education in England. In P. Lang, Y. Katz, & I. Menezes (Eds.), *Affective education: A comparative view* (pp. 72–83). London: Cassell.

Bevis, E. O., & Watson, J. (1989*). Toward a caring curriculum: A new pedagogy for nursing.* New York, NY: National League for Nursing Press.

Bilchik, G. (2002). A better place to heal. *Health Forum Journal, 45*(4), 10–15.

Billings, D., & Halstead, J. (2009). *Teaching in nursing: A guide for faculty (*3rd ed.). St. Louis, MO: Saunders.

Billings, D., & Halstead, J. (2012). *Teaching in nursing: A guide for faculty (*4th ed.). St. Louis, MO: Elsevier Saunders.

Bingham, C., & Sidorkin, A. M. (Eds.). (2004). *No education without relation.* New York, NY: Peter Lang Publishing, Inc.

Blakely, G., Skirton, H., Cooper, S., Allum, P., & Nelmes, P. (2009). Educational gaming in the health sciences: Systematic review. *Journal of Advanced Nursing, 65*(2); 259–269.

Blakemore, C., & Cooper, G. F. (1970). Development of the brain depends on the visual environment. *Nature, 228*, 477–478.

Bly, R. (1988). *A little book on the human shadow.* San Francisco, CA: Harper and Row Publishers.

Boyatzis, R., Goleman, D., & Rhee, K. (2000). Clustering competence in emotional intelligence: Insights from the emotional competence inventory (ECI). In J. R. Bar-On & D. A. Parker (Eds.), *Handbook of emotional intelligence* (pp. 343–362). San Francisco, CA: Jossey-Bass.

Boyatzis, R., & Van Oosten, E. (2002). Developing emotional intelligent organizations. In R. Millar (Ed.), *International executive development programmes* (7th ed.). London: Kogan Page Publishers.

Boyer, E. (1987). *College: The undergraduate experience in America.* New York, NY: Harper and Row.

Boyer, E. (1990). *Scholarship reconsidered: Priorities of the professorate.* Princeton, NJ: Carnegie Foundation for the Advancement of Teaching.

Bradshaw, A. (1998). Charting some challenges in the art and science of nursing. *The Lancet, 351*(9100), 438–440.

Brookfield, S. D. (1995). *Becoming a critically reflective teacher.* San Francisco, CA: Jossey-Bass.

Burns, N., & Grove, S. K. (2008). *The practice of nursing research: Appraisal, synthesis, and generation of Evidence* (6th ed.). Philadelphia, PA: W. B. Saunders Company.

Callan, E. (1997/2004). *Creating citizens: Political education and liberal democracy.* Oxford, UK: Oxford University Press.

Carper, B. A. (1978). Fundamental patterns of knowing in nursing. *Advances in Nursing Science, 1*(1), 12–23.

Chavez, M. (1994, November 18–20). *Learners' perspectives on authenticity.* A paper presented at the American Council on the Teaching of Foreign Languages, Atlanta, GA.

Cherniss, C. (2000). *Emotional intelligence: What it is and why it matters.* Paper presented at the annual meeting of the Society for Industrial and Organizational Psychology, New Orleans, LA. Retrieved April, 2000, from www.eiconsortium.org

Cherniss, C., & Goleman, D. (1998). *Bringing emotional intelligence to the workplace.* A technical report issued by the Consortium for Research on Emotional Intelligence in Organizations. Retrieved October 7, 1998, from www.eiconsortium.org

Clark, R. (1994). Media will never influence learning. *Educational Technology Research and Development, 42*(2), 21–30.

Clark, R., & Choi, S. (2007). The questionable benefits of pedagogical agents: Response to Veletsianos. *Journal of Educational Computing Research, 36*(4), 379–381.

Clark, R., & Mayer, R. (2008). *E-learning and the science of instruction: Proven guidelines for consumers and designers of multimedia learning.* San Francisco, CA: Pfeiffer.

Clark, R. E. (2009). Resistance to change: Unconscious knowledge and the challenge of unlearning. In D. C. Berliner & Haggai Kupermintz (Eds.), *Fostering change in institutions, environments, and people* (pp. 75–94). New York, NY: Routledge.

Cohen, J. (2001). Social and emotional education: Core concepts and practices. In J. Cohen (Ed.), *Caring classrooms, intelligent schools: The social emotional education of young children* (pp. 3–29). New York, NY: Teachers College Press.

Cohen, J. (2006). Social, emotional, ethical, and academic education: Creating a climate for learning, participation in democracy and well-being. *Harvard Educational Review,* 76(2), 201–237.

Collier, J., & Collier, M. (1986). *Visual anthropology: Photography as a research method.* Albuquerque, NM: University of New Mexico Press.

Collins, U. (1998). Fiche bliain ag fas (Twenty years a-growing). In P. Lang, Y. Katz, & I. Menezes (Eds.), *Affective education: A comparative view* (pp. 36–45). London: Cassell.

Conan, N. (2012, September 24). *Many of us are small stakes cheaters, but why? Talk of the Nation* on NPR radio broadcast. Retrieved from http://www.npr.org/2012/09/24/161696134/many-of-us-are-small-stakes-cheaters-but-why

Conrad, C. F. (1989, Spring). Meditations on the ideology of inquiry in higher education: Exposition, critique, and conjecture. *The Review of Higher Education, 12*(3), 199–220.

Conrad, R., & Donaldson, J. (2004). *Engaging the online learner: Activities and resources for creative instruction.* San Francisco, CA: Jossey-Bass.

Cooper, R. (1997). *Executive EQ: Emotional intelligence in leadership and organizations.* New York, NY: Grosset and Putnam.

Cornelius-White, J. (2007, March). Learner-centered teacher–student relationships are effective: A meta-analysis. *Review of Educational Research,* 77(1), 113–143.

Corsini, R. J., & Wedding, D. (Eds.). (2011). *Current psychotherapies* (9th ed.). Belmont, CA: F.E. Brooks/Cole.

Crossley, N. (1996). *Intersubjectivity: The fabric of social becoming.* Thousand Oaks, CA: Sage Publications.

Cuthbert, P. F. (2005). The student learning process: Learning styles of learning approaches? *Teaching in Higher Education, 10*(2), 235–249.

Darder, A. (2002). *Reinventing Paulo Freire: A pedagogy of love.* Boulder, CO: Westview Press.

Davis, J. R. (1993). *Better teaching, more learning: Strategies for success in postsecondary settings.* Phoenix, AZ: Oryx Press.

Day, C. (2004). *A passion for teaching.* New York, NY: RoutledgeFalmer.

Dayton, T. (1994). *The drama within: Psychodrama and experiential therapy.* Deerfield Beach, FL: Health Communications, Inc.

Deci, E.L., & Flaste, R. (1995). *Why we do what we do.* New York, NY: G.P. Putnam's Sons.

Dede, Y. (2009). The contribution of the comprehension tests to the cognitive and affective development of prospective teachers: A case study. *The Montana Mathematics Enthusiast, 6*(3), 497–526.

Denzin, N. K., & Lincoln, Y. S. (2000). (Eds.) *Handbook of qualitative research.* Thousand Oaks, CA: Sage Publishing.

Dewey, J. (1944/1916). *Democracy and education.* New York, NY: The Free Press.

Dipietro, M., Ferdig, R., Boyer, J., & Black, E. (2007). Towards a framework for understanding electronic educational gaming. *Journal of Educational Multimedia & Hypermedia, 16*(3), 225–248.

Dispenza, J. (2005). In W. Arntz, B. Chasse, & M. Vicente (2005). *What the bleep do we know: Discovering the endless possibilities for altering your everyday reality,* p. 55. Deerfield Beach, CA: Health Communications, Inc.

Downing, C. (Ed.). (1991). *Mirrors of the self.* Los Angeles, CA: Jeremy P. Tarcher, Inc.

Dreesmann, H. (1982). Unterichtsklima: wie Schuler den Unterricht wahrnehmen, Bwinheim: Beltz Verlag. In Fess, R. (1998). *Affective education in Germany. Existing structures and opportunities: Are we using them effectively?* In P. Lang, Y. Katz, & I. Menezes (Eds.), *Affective education: A comparative view* (pp. 28–35). London: Cassell.

Duffy, J. (1990). *The relationship between nurse caring behaviors and selected outcomes of care in hospitalized medical and/or surgical patients.* Unpublished doctoral dissertation. Washington, DC: Catholic University of America.

Einstein, A. (n.d.) Found in L. Secretan (2004). *Inspire: What great leaders do.* Hoboken, NJ: John Wiley & Sons, Inc.

Elias, M. J. (2006). The connection between academic and social-emotional learning. In M. J. Elias & H. Arnold (Eds.), *The educator's guide to emotional intelligence and academic achievement: Social emotional learning in the classroom* (pp. 4–44). Thousand Oaks, CA: Corwin Press.

Elias, M. J. (2009, November). Social-emotional and character development and academics as a dula focus of educational policy. *Education Policy, 23*(6), 831–846.

Elias, M. J., Zins, J. E., Weissberg, R. P., Forey, K. S., Greenberg, M. T., Haynes, N. M., et al. (1997). *Promoting social and emotional learning: Guidelines for educators.* Alexandria, VA: Association for Supervision and Curriculum Development.

Ellis, R. (1989). Rational-emotive therapy. In R. J. Corsini and D. Wedding (Eds.), *Current psychotherapies* (4th ed.) (pp. 197–240). Itasca, IL: F.E. Peacock Publishers, Inc.

Emoto, M. (2004). *The hidden messages in water.* Hillsboro, OR: Beyond Words Publishing, Inc. Retrieved from http://www.youtube.com/watch?v=33IiYb8htHk&feature=youtu.be

Escher, M. C. (2000). *The magic of M. C. Escher.* New York, NY: Harry N. Abrams, Inc. and http://www.mcescher.com/Biography/biography.htm

Fawcett, J. (1995). *Analysis and evaluations of conceptual models of Nursing* (3rd ed.). Philadelphia, PA: F. A. Davis Company.

Felgen, J. (2004). A caring and healing environment. In M. Koloroutis (Ed.), *Relationship-based care: A model for transforming practice* (pp. 23–52). Minneapolis, MN: Creative Healthcare Management.

Fess, R. (1998). *Affective education in Germany. Existing structures and opportunities: Are we using them effectively?* In P. Lang, Y. Katz, & I. Menezes (Eds.), *Affective education: A comparative view* (pp. 28–35). London: Cassell.

Finke, L. M., (2009). Teaching in nursing: The faculty role. In D. M. Billings & J. A. Halstead (3rd ed.), *Teaching in nursing: A guide for faculty* (pp. 3–17). St. Louis, MO: Saunders-Elsevier.

Fleming, G. (n.d.). Cheating with technology: It's still cheating! About.com Homework /Study Tips (a NY Times Company). Retrieved on August 31, 2012, from http://homeworktips.about.com/of/cheating/a/echeating.htm

Flew, A. (1984) *A dictionary of philosophy.* New York, NY: St. Martin's Press.

Ford, D. (2002). *The secret of the shadow.* San Francisco, CA: Harper.

Ford, D. (2010). *The dark side of the light chaser.* New York, NY: Riverhead Books.

Fox, J. (1987). *The essential Moreno.* New York, NY: Springer Publishing Company.

Fraser, B. J., Wahlberg, H. J., Welch, W. W., & Hattie, J. A. (1987). Syntheses of educational productivity research. *International Journal of Educational Research, 11*, 144–252.

Freire, P. (1970/2009). *Pedagogy of the oppressed.* New York, NY: Continuum.

Freire, P. (1998). *Teachers as cultural workers: Letters to those who dare to teach.* Boulder, CO: Westview.

Frymier, A. B. (1993, Fall). The impact of teacher immediacy on students' motivation: Is it the same for all students? *Communication Quarterly, 41*(4), 453–464.

Frymier, A. B. (1994, Spring). A model of immediacy in the classroom. *Communication Quarterly, 42*(2), 133–144.

Frymier, A. B., & Schulman, G. M. (1994, November 19–22). *Development and testing of the learner empowerment instrument in a communication based model.* Paper presented at the annual meeting of the Speech Communication Association in New Orleans, LA.

Gaut, D. A. (1992). *The presence of caring in nursing.* New York, NY: National League for Nursing Press.

Gigerenzer, G. (2007). *Gut feeling: The intelligence of the unconscious.* New York, NY: Viking-Penguin Books.

Gilje, F. (1992). Being there: An analysis of the concept of presence. In D. Gaut (Ed.), *The presence of caring in nursing* (pp. 53–67). New York, NY: National League for Nursing Press.

Glesne, C., & Peshkin, A. (1992). *Becoming qualitative researchers: An introduction.* New York: Longman

Goleman, D. (1995). *Emotional intelligence: Why it can matter more than IQ.* New York, NY: Bantam Books.

Goleman, D. (1998). *Working with emotional intelligence.* New York, NY: Bantam Books.

Goleman, D. (2006). *Social intelligence: The new science of human relations.* New York, NY: Bantam Books.

Gorham, J. (1988, January). The relationship between verbal teacher immediacy behaviors and student learning. *Communication Education, 37,* 40–53.

Graczyk, P. A., Weissberg, R. P., Payton, J. W., Elias, M. J., Greenberg, M. T., and Zins, J. E. (2000). Criteria for evaluating the quality of school-based social and emotional learning programs. In R. Bar-On & J. D. Parker (Eds.), *Handbook of emotional intelligence: Theory development, assessment, and application at home, school and in the workplace* (pp. 391–410). San Francisco, CA: Jossey-Bass.

Greene, J. C. (1994). Qualitative program evaluation: Practice and promise. In N. Y. Denzin & Y. S. Lincoln (Eds.), *Handbook of qualitative research* (pp. 530–544). Newbury Park, CA: Sage Publications.

Hagedorn, M. (1990). Using photography with families of chronically ill children. In M. Leininger & J. Watson (Eds.), *The caring imperative in education* (pp. 227–235). New York: National League for Nursing.

Hall, C. S., & Nordby, V. J. (1973). *A primer of Jungian psychology.* New York, NY: Mentor Books.

Halldorsdottir, S. (1990). The essential structure of a caring and an uncaring encounter with teacher: The perspective of the nursing student. In M. Leininger & J. Watson (Eds.), *The caring imperative in education* (pp. 95–109). New York, NY: National League for Nursing.

Halldorsdottir, S. (1991). Five basic modes of being with another. In D. A. Gaut and M. Leininger (Eds.), *Caring: The compassionate healer* (pp. 37–50). New York, NY: National League for Nursing.

Halstead, J. A. (2007). *Nurse educator competencies: Creating an evidence-based practice for nurse educators.* New York, NY: National League for Nursing.

Hammer, E. (1990). *Reaching the affect.* Northvale, NJ: Jason Aronson, Inc.

Hardy, R. E. (1991). *Gestalt psychotherapy: Concepts and demonstrations in stress, relationships, hypnosis, and addiction.* Springfield, IL: Charles C. Thomas Publishers.

Harrison, E. (1995). Nurse caring and the new health care paradigm. *Journal of Nursing Care Quality, 9*(4), 14–23.

Hativa, N., & Birenbaum, M. (2000). Who prefers what? Disciplinary differences in students' preferred approaches to teaching and learning styles. *Research in Higher Education, 41*(2) 209–236.

Hattie, J. A. (1999, August 2). *Influences on student learning.* Inaugural lecture, University of Auckland, New Zealand.

Hays, L. (2010). *The eyes have it . . . the caring moment: One nurse to another.* Presented at Exempla Lutheran Medical Center as part of the Model of Care presentation.

Heidbreder, E. (1933). *Seven psychologies.* New York, NY: Appleton Century Crofts, Inc.

Heidegger, M. (1962). *Being and time.* New York, NY: Harper and Row Publishers.

Henry, J. (1997). Gaming: A teaching strategy to enhance adult learning. *Journal of Continuing Education in Nursing, 28*(5); 231–234.

Heshusius, L. (1994, April). Freeing ourselves from objectivity: Managing subjectivity or turning toward a participatory mode of consciousness? *Educational Researcher, 23*(3), 15–22.

Hoffman, D. M. (2009, June). Reflecting on social emotional learning: A critical perspective on trends in the United States. *Review of Educational Research, 79*(2), 533–556.

Hooks, B. (1999). Embracing freedom: Spirituality and liberation. In S. Glazer (Ed.), *The heart of learning: Spirituality in education* (pp. 113–129). New York, NY: Penguin Putnam Inc.

Horgan, J. (1992, July). Quantum philosophy. Published in 1992 in *Scientific American* posted on a web page in 2002. Retrieved 5/31/2011 from www.fortunecity.com/emachines/e11/86/qphil.html

Hughes, L. (1995, May/June). Teaching caring to nursing students. *Nurse Educator, 20*(3), 3–4.

IANS. (2012, August 31). Harvard probes dozens of students on cheating allegation. *Yahoo! News.* Retrieved from http://in.news.yahoo.com/harvard-probes-dozens-students-cheating-allegation-063314734.html

Jacobi, J. (1973). *The psychology of C. G. Jung.* New Haven, CT: Yale University Press.

Jacobs-Kramer, M. K., & Chinn, P. L. (1992). Perspectives on knowing: A model of nursing knowledge. In L. H. Nicoll (Ed.), *Perspectives on nursing theory* (2nd ed.; pp. 289–296). Philadelphia, PA: J. B. Lippincott Company.

Jahn, R. G., & Dunne, B. J. (1997). Science of the subjective, *Journal of Scientific Exploration, 11*(2), 201–224.

Jung, C. G. (1933). *A modern man in search of a soul.* New York, NY: Harcourt Brace Jovanovich.

Kaku, M. (2011). *Physics of the future: How science will shape human destiny and our daily lives by the year 2100.* New York, NY: Doubleday.

Kaplan, C., & Schrecker, E. (1983). *Regulating the intellectuals: Perspectives on academic freedom in the 1980s.* New York, NY: Praeger Publishing.

Karl, J. (1992). Being there: Who do you bring to practice? In D. A. Gaut (Ed.), *The presence of caring in nursing* (pp. 1–13). New York, NY: National League for Nursing Press.

Kellerman, P. F. (1979). Transference, counter-transference and tele. *Journal of Group Psychotherapy, Psychodrama and Sociometry, 32*, 38–55.

Kennedy, D. (1990, April). President of Stanford University. Speech presented to the faculty, April 1990.

Kiegaldie, D., & White, G. (2006). The virtual patient—Development, implementation and evaluation of an innovative computer simulation for postgraduate nursing students. *Journal of Educational Multimedia and Hypermedia, 15*(17), 31.

Kimble, C., Hildreth, P., & Bourdon, I. (Eds.). (2008). *Communities of practice: Creating learning environments for educators,* vol. 1. Charlotte, NC: Information Age Publishing, Inc.

King, E. C. (1984). *Affective education in nursing: A guide to teaching and assessment.* Rockville, MD: Aspen.

King, I. M. (1971). *Toward a theory for nursing: General concepts of human behavior.* New York, NY: John Wiley & Sons, Inc.

Kirman, W. J. (1977) *Modern psychoanalysis in the schools.* Wayne, NJ: Avery Publishing Group, Inc.

Klimek, M. (1990). Virtue, ethics, and care: Developing the personal dimensions of caring in nursing education. In M. Leininger & J. Watson (Eds.), *The caring imperative in education* (pp. 177–189). New York: National League for Nursing.

Koerner, J. G. (2007). *Healing presence: The essence of nursing.* New York, NY: Springer Publishing Company.

Koloroutis, M. (Ed.). (2004). *Relationship-based care: A model for transforming practice.* Minneapolis, MN: Creative Health Care Management.

Krathwohl, D. R., Bloom, B. S., & Masia, B. B. (1964/1974/1999). *Taxonomy of educational objectives: The classification of educational goals* (Handbook II: Affective domain). New York, NY: David McKay Company, Inc. (1999 edition published by Longman.)

Kushnir, L. (2009). When knowing more means knowing less: Understanding the impact of computer experience on e-learning and e-learning outcomes. *Electronic Journal of e-Learning,* 7(3) 289–299.

Lang, P. (1998). Toward an understanding of affective education in a European context. In P. Lang, Y. Katz, & I. Menezes (Eds.), *Affective education: A comparative view* (pp. 3–16). London: Cassell.

Lang, P., Katz, Y., & Menezes, I. (Eds.). (1998). *Affective education: A comparative view.* London: Cassell.

Lasater, K. (2007). Clinical judgment development: Using simulation to create an assessment rubric. *Journal of Nursing Education, 46*(11), 496–503.

Lave, J., & Wenger, E. (1998). Communities of practice. Retrieved 10/12/2012 from http://www.learning-theories.com/communities-of-practice-lave-and-wenger.html

Lean, J., Moizer, J., Towler, M., & Abbey, C. (2006). Simulations and games: Use and barriers in higher education. *Active Learning in Higher Education,* 7(3), 227–242.

Leatherman, C. (1996, November 1). Appeals court reverses ruling that University of Minnesota limited professors' free speech. *Chronicle of Higher Education, XLIII*(10), A11–A12.

Leininger, M. M. (1984). *Care: An essential human need.* Thorofare, NJ: Slack.

Leininger, M. M., & Watson, J. (1990). *The caring imperative in education.* New York, NY: National League for Nursing.

Leslie, D. W., & Beckham, J. C. (1986, Winter). Research on higher education: Dead end or new directions? *The Review of Higher Education, 10*(2), 123–128.

Likert, R. (1932). Techniques for the measurement of attitudes. In *Archives of psychology 22*(140), pp. 1–55.

Lincoln, Y. S., & Guba, E. G. (1985). *Naturalistic inquiry.* Newbury Park, CA: Sage Publications.

Lowman, J. (1995). *What constitutes masterful teaching?: Mastering the techniques of teaching.* San Francisco, CA: Josey-Bass.

Lucas, C. J. (1996). *Crisis in the academy: Rethinking higher education in America.* New York: St. Martin's Press.

Lysaught, J. P. (1970). *An abstract for action.* New York, NY: McGraw-Hill.

Malkin, J. (1992). *Hospital interior architecture.* Hoboken, NJ: John Wiley & Sons.

Mather, J. A., & Champagne, A. (Spring, 2008). Student learning styles/strategies and professors' expectations: Do they match? *College Quarterly, 11*(2). Retrieved from www.collegequarterly.ca/2008-vol11-num02-spring/mather-champagne.html

Mayerhoff, M. (1970). *On caring.* New York, NY: Harper and Row.

Mayes, C. (2003). *Seven curricular landscapes: An approach to the holistic curriculum.* New York, NY: University Press of America, Inc. (56, 59).

Mayo, C. (2004). Relations are difficult. In C. Bingham & A. M. Sidorkin (Eds.), *No education without relation* (pp. 121–135). New York, NY: Peter Lang Publishing, Inc.

McConnell, T. R. (1987). Autonomy and accountability: Some fundamental issues. In P. G. Altbach & R. O. Berdahl (Eds.), *Higher education in American society* (pp. 39–58). Buffalo, NY: Prometheus Books.

McFarlane, T. J. (1995). Quantum mechanics and reality. Retrieved at www.integralscience.org

McTaggart, L. (2007). *The intention experiment: Using your thoughts to change your life and the world.* New York, NY: Free Press.

Milić, M., & Škorić, I. (2010). The impact of formal education on computer literacy. *International Journal of Emerging Technologies in Learning, 5*, 60–63.

Miller, B. K., Haber, J., & Byrne, M. W. (1992). The experience of caring in the acute care setting: Patient and nurse perspectives. In D. A. Gaut (Ed.), *The presence of caring in nursing* (pp. 137–156). New York, NY: National League for Nursing Press.

Montgomery, C. L. (1992). The spiritual connection: Nurses' perceptions of the experience of caring. In D. A. Gaut (Ed.), *The presence of caring in nursing* (pp. 39–52). New York, NY: National League for Nursing Press.

Moore, A. (1996, January). College teacher immediacy and student rating of instructors. *Communication Education, 45*, 29–39.

Moore, T. (1992/1940). *Care of the soul: A guide for cultivating depth and sacredness in everyday life.* New York, NY: Harper Collins Publishers.

Moreno, J. L. (1953). *Who shall survive?* New York, NY: Beacon House.

Moussly, R. (2012, August 18). Student cheating is a serious problem in the UAE, academic says. *Gulfnews.com*. Retrieved from http://gulfnews.com/news/gulf/uae/education/student-cheating-is-a-serious-problem-in-the-uae-academic-says-1.1061287

Muchmore, J. (n.d.). PowerPoint etiquette. Retrieved September 22, 2012, from http://www.muchmorebi.com/powerpoint_etiquette.htm

Munhall, P. (1993, May/June). Unknowing: Toward another pattern of knowing in nursing. *Nursing Outlook, 41*, 125–128.

Muszynski, H. (1977). In P. Lang, Y. Katz, & I. Menezes (Eds.), *Affective education: A comparative view* (p. 11). London: Cassell.

Napier, N. J. (1990). *Re-creating your self.* New York, NY: W. W. Norton & Company.

National League for Nursing. (2003). *Innovation in nursing education: A call to reform—Position statement.* National League of Nursing, Board of Governors. Retrieved from http://www.nln.org/aboutnln/PositionStatements/innovation082203.pdf

National League for Nursing (2005). *Core competencies of nursing educators with task statements.* Retrieved February 5, 2010, from http://www.nln.org/facultydevelopment/pdf/corecompetencies.pdf

National League for Nursing. (2005). *Transforming nursing education—Position Statement.* National League of Nursing, Board of Governors. Retrieved from http://www.nln.org/aboutnln/PositionStatements/transforming052005.pdf

National Research Council (NRC). (2000). *Digital dilemma: Intellectual property in the information age*. Washington, DC: National Academies Press. Retrieved from http://www.nap.edu/catalog/9601.html

Neville, C. (2007). *Complete guide to referencing and avoiding plagiarism*. Berkshire, England: Open University Press.

Newberg, A. (2005). In W. Arntz, B. Chasse, & M. Vicente (2005). *What the bleep do we know: Discovering the endless possibilities for altering your everyday reality* (p. 54). Deerfield Beach, CA: Health Communications, Inc.

Nodding, N. (2005). *The challenge to care in schools: An alternative approach to education* (2nd ed.). New York, NY: Teachers College Press.

Nodding, N. (2006). Education whole people: A response to Jonathan Cohen. *Harvard Educational Review, 76*(2), 238–242.

O'Brien, D. (1986). The university as a place of learning. *Liberal Education, 72*(2), 139–144.

Olswang, S. G., & Lee, B. A. (1984). *Faculty freedoms and institutional accountability: Interactions and conflicts*. Washington, DC: Association for the Study of Higher Education.

Ondrejka, D. (1998). *Affective pedagogy in higher education* (Doctoral dissertation). [Microfilm]. Ann Arbor, MI: University Microfilms International, 1999.

O'Neil, R. M. (1996, September 13). Protecting free speech when the issue is sexual harassment. *Chronicle of Higher Education, 43*(3), B3–B4.

Orem, D. E. (1971). *Nursing concepts of practice*. New York, NY: McGraw-Hill Book Company.

Ornstein, A. C. (1995, Winter). The new paradigm in research on teaching. *The Educational Forum, 59*, 124–129.

Palloff, R., & Pratt, K. (2011). *The excellent online instructor*. San Francisco, CA: Jossey-Bass.

Palmer, P. (1999). The grace of great things: Reclaiming the sacred in knowing, teaching, and learning. In S. Glazer (Ed.), *The heart of learning: Spirituality in education* (pp. 23–29). New York, NY: Jeremy P. Tarcher/Putnam.

Palmer, P. (2004). *A hidden wholeness: The journey toward an undivided life*. San Francisco, CA: Jossey-Bass.

Palmer, P. (2007). *The courage to teach: Exploring the inner landscape of a teaching life* (10th Anniversary ed.). San Francisco, CA: Jossey-Bass.

Pampliega, A. M., & Marroquin, M. (1998). Affective education and the new Spanish educational reforms. In P. Lang, Y. Katz, & I. Menezes (Eds.), *Affective education: A comparative view* (pp. 85–98). London: Cassell.

Paradi, D. (2010, February 15). *102 tips to improve how to use PowerPoint*. Mississauga, Ontario, Canada: Self-published. Retrieved from http://pptideas.blogspot.com/2010/03/new-book-102-tips-to-communicate-more.html

Pardue, K., Tagliareni, M., & Valiga, T. (2005, Jan/Feb). Substantive innovation in nursing education: Shifting the emphasis from content coverage to student learning. *Nursing Education Perspectives, 26*(1), 55–57.

Pearson, K. (1911/2007). *The grammar of science*. New York, NY: Cosimo, Inc.

Perls, F. (1969). *Gestalt therapy verbatim*. Lafayette, CA: Real People Press.

Perls, F. (1972). *In and out of the garbage pail*. New York, NY: Bantam Books.

Pert, C. (2005). Sight and perception. In W. Arntz, B. Chasse, & M. Vicente (2005). *What the bleep do we know: Discovering the endless possibilities for altering your everyday reality* (p. 54). Deerfield Beach, CA: Health Communications, Inc.

Peterson, M. (1986, Winter). Critical choices: From adolescence to maturity in higher education research. *The Review of Higher Education, 10*(2), 143–150.

Piane, G., Rydman, R. J., & Rudens. A. J. (1996). Learning style preferences of public health students. *Journal of Medical Systems, 20*(6), 377–384.

Polkinghorne, D. (1983). *Methodology for the human sciences: Systems of inquiry*. Albany, NY: State University of New York Press.

Prus, R. (1996). *Symbolic interaction and ethnographic research*. Albany, NY: State University of New York Press.

Remen, N. R. (1996). *Kitchen table wisdom: Stories that heal*. New York, NY: Riverhead Books.

Remen, N. R. (1999). Education for mission, meaning and compassion. In S. Glazer (Ed.) *The heart of learning: Spirituality in education* (pp. 33–50). New York, NY: Penguin Putnam, Inc.

Richardson, L. (1994). Writing: A method of inquiry. In N. Y. Denzin & Y. S. Lincoln (Eds.), *Handbook of qualitative research* (pp. 516–529). Newbury Park, CA: Sage Publications.

Roach, M. S. (1992). Response to: Being there: Who do you bring to practice? In D. A. Gaut (Ed.), *The presence of caring in nursing* (pp. 14–23). New York, NY: National League for Nursing Press.

Robinson, R. Y. (1995, May 25–29). *Affiliative communication behaviors: A comparative analysis of the interrelationships among teacher nonverbal immediacy, responsiveness, and verbal receptivity on the prediction of student learning*. Paper presentation at the International Communication Association in Albuquerque, NM.

Roblyer, M. (2006). *Integrating educational technology into teaching*. Upper Saddle River, NJ: Prentice Hall, Inc.

Roblyer, M., & Doering, A. (2010). *Integrating educational technology into teaching*. Upper Saddle River, NJ: Pearson Education, Inc.

Rogers, C. R. (1951). *Client centered therapy*. London: Constable

Rogers, C. R. (1961). *On becoming a person: A therapist's view of psychotherapy*. Boston, MA: Houghton Mifflin.

Rogers, C. R. (1969). *Freedom to learn*. Columbus, OH: Charles E. Merral.

Rogers, M. (1970). *The theoretical basis of nursing*. Philadelphia, PA: F. A. Davis Company.

Rosenblum, B., & Kuttner, F. (2006). *Quantum enigma: Physics encounters consciousness*. New York, NY: Oxford University Press.

Rotheram-Boris, M. J., & Tesembaris, S. J. (1989). Social competency training programs in ethnically diverse communities. In L. Bond & C. Swift (Eds.), *Primary prevention and promotion in the schools* (pp. 297–318). Newbury Park, CA: Sage.

Roy, Sr. C. (1976). *Introduction to nursing: An adaptation model.* Englewood Cliffs, NJ: Prentice-Hall, Inc.

Royse, M., & Newton, S. (2007). How gaming is used as an innovative strategy for nursing education. *Nursing Education Perspectives, 28*(5), 263–267.

Ruiz, D. M. (1999). *The mastery of love.* San Rafael, CA: Amber-Allen Publishing.

Ruiz, M. (1997). *The four agreements: A practical guide.* San Rafael, CA: Amber-Allen Publishing.

Salovey, P., & Mayer, J. D. (1990). Emotional intelligence. *Imagination, Cognition, and Personality, 9*, 185–211.

Samaras, A. P., Freese, A. R., Kosnik, C., & Beck, C. (Eds.). (2008). *Learning communites in practice.* New York, NY: Springer Publishing Company.

Sauvé, L., Renaud, L., Kaufman, D., & Marquis, J. (2007). Distinguishing between games and simulations: A systematic review. *Educational Technology & Society, 10*(3), 247–256.

Schiavenato, M. (2009). Reevaluating simulation in nursing education: Beyond the human patient simulator. *Journal of Nursing Education, 48*(7), 388–394.

Schoenly, L. (1994). Teaching in the affective domain. *The Journal of Continuing Education in Nursing, 25*(5), 209–212.

Schunk, D. (2012). *Learning theories: An educational perspective* (6th ed.). Upper Saddle River, NJ: Pearson Education, Inc.

Secretan, L. (2004). *Inspire: What great leaders do.* Hoboken, NJ: John Wiley & Sons, Inc.

Shen, L., Wang, M., & Shen, R. (2009). Affective e-learning: Using "emotional" data to improve learning in pervasive learning environments. *Educational Technology & Society, 12*(2), 176–189.

Silverman, M. P. (2010). *Quantum superposition: Counterintuitive, consequences of coherence, entanglement, and interference.* Verlag Berlin Heidlberg: Springer.

Simons, D., & Chabris, C. (1999). *Selective attentiveness test.* Retrieved from http://www.youtube.com/watch?v=vJG698U2Mvo&feature=youtu.be

Singham, M. (2007). Death to the syllabus. *Liberal Education, 93*(4), 52–56.

Slate, J. (2002). *Psychic vampires: Protection from energy predators and parasites.* St. Paul, MN: Llewellyn Publications.

Slaughter, S. (1987). Academic freedom in the modern university. In P. G. Altbach & R. O. Berdahl (Eds.), *Higher education in American society* (pp. 77–106). Buffalo, NY: Prometheus Books.

Spitzberg, I. J. (1987). It's academic: The politics of the curriculum. In P. G. Altbach and R. O. Berdahl (Eds.), *Higher education in American society* (pp. 297–311). Buffalo, NY: Prometheus Books.

Steiner, C. (1997). *Achieving emotional literacy*. New York, NY: Avon Books.

Steiner, R. (2008/1947). *Knowledge of the higher worlds and their attainment*. Radford, VA: Wilder Publishing, LLC.

Stern, R. (2007). Social and emotional learning: What is it? How can we use it to help our children? Retrieved from http://www.aboutourkids.org/articles/social_emotional_learning_what_it_how_can_we_use_it_help_our_children

Thayer-Bacon, B. (2004). Personal and social relations in education. In C. Bingham & A. M. Sidorkin (Eds.), *No education without relation* (pp. 165–179). New York, NY: Peter Lang Publishing, Inc.

TIGER. (2007–2010). *Technology informatics guiding educational reform*. Retrieved on November 11, 2010, from http://www.tigersummit.com/About_Us.html

Tuckman, B. W. (1965). Developmental sequence in small groups. *Psychological Bulletin, 63*, 384–399.

Tyler, R. (1949). *Basic principles of curriculum and instruction*. Chicago, IL: The University of Chicago Press.

Ulrich, R. (1984). View through a window may influence recovery from surgery. *Science, 224*(4647), 420–421.

Vermunt, J. D., & Vermetten, Y. J. (2004). Patterns in student learning: Relationships between learning strategies, conceptions of learning, and learning orientation. *Educational Psychology Review, 16*(4), 359–384.

Washington Center for Nursing. (2009). A master plan for nursing education in Washington state: Implementation recommendations. (Changed from innovation workgroup briefing paper to a master plan.) Retrieved from http://www.wacenterfornursing.org/uploads/file/nursing-education/mpne-implementation-recommendations-12-09.pdf

Watkins, R. (2005). *75 e-learning activities: Making online learning interactive*. San Francisco, CA: Pfeiffer.

Watson, J. (1979). *Nursing: The philosophy and science of caring*. Boulder, CO: University Press of Colorado.

Watson, J. (1981). Some issues related to a science of caring for nursing practice. In M. M. Leininger (Ed.), *Caring: A human helping process* (pp. 23–40). Thorofare, NJ: Slack.

Watson, J. (1985). *Human science and human care*. Norwalk, CT: Appleton-Century-Crofts.

Watson, J. (1988). Human caring as moral context for nursing education. *Nursing & Health Care, 9*, 423–425.

Watson, J. (1989). Watson's philosophy and theory of human caring in nursing. In J. Riehl-Sisca (Ed.), *Conceptual models for nursing practice* (3rd ed.) (pp. 219–236). Norwalk, CT: Appleton & Lange.

Watson, J. (2004). Forward. In M. Koloratous (Ed.), *Relationship based care: A model for transforming practice* (p. viii). Minneapolis, MN: Creative Health Care Management.

Watson, J. (2008). *Nursing: The philosophy and science of caring* (Rev. ed.). Boulder, CO: University Press of Colorado.

Weimer, M. (2010). *Inspired college teaching: A career-long resource for professional growth*. San Francisco, CA: Jossey-Bass.

Weisinger, H. (1997). *Emotional intelligence at work: The untapped edge for success.* San Francisco, CA: Jossey-Bass Publishers.

What the bleep do we know?: Down the rabbit hole. Copyright, 2004 by Lord of the Wind Films, LLC. Distributed by Captured Light Distributions at www.whatthebleep.com. [Interviewed physicists: William Tiller, Amit Goswami, John Hagelin, Fred Alan Wolf, and David Albert. Interviewed neurologists, anesthesiologists, and physicians: Masaru Emoto, Stuart Hameroff, Andrew Newberg, Jeffrey Satinover, Daniel Monti, and Joseph Dispenza. Interviewed molecular biologist: Candace Pert. Interviewed spiritual scholar and teacher: Ramtha and Miceal Ledwith.

Whitfield, C. L. (1987). *The child within: Discovery and recovery for adult children of dysfunctional families.* Deerfield Beach, FL: Health Communications, Inc.

Wilber, K. 2000. *Integral psychology: Consciousness, spirit, psychology, therapy.* Boston, MA: Shambhala.

Williams, A. (1989). *The passionate technique: Strategic psychodrama with individuals, families, and groups.* New York, NY: Tavistock/Routledge.

Williamson, M. (1992). *A return to love: Reflections on the principles of a course in miracles.* New York, NY: HarperCollins Publishing.

Williamson, M. (n.d.). Our deepest fear. (Provided to Nelson Mandela for his inaugural speech.) Retrieved from http://thinkexist.com/quotes/marianne_williamson/

Wilson, R. (1997, December 12). Professor faces harassment charge for disclaimer about 'adult themes' in his class. *The Chronicle of Higher Education, XLIV*(16), A14.

Woods, J. H. (1993). Affective learning: One door to critical thinking. *Holistic Nursing Practice,* 7(3), 64–70.

Wolfe, K., Bates, D., Manikowske, L., & Amundsen, R. (2006). Learning styles: Do they differ by discipline. *Journal of Family and Consumer Sciences, 9*(4), 18–22.

Wulff, D. H., & Austin, A. E. (2004). *Paths to the professoriate: Strategies for enriching the preparation of future faculty.* San Francisco, CA: Jossey-Bass.

Yaccino, S. (2008, October 3). Cheating students use technology, too. *U.S. News & World Report, LP.* Retrieved from www.usnews.com/education/articles/2008/10/03/cheating-students-use-technology-too

Yanovasky, V. S. (1978). *Medicine, science and life.* New York, NY: Paulist Press.

YouTube. (2010, November 23). Cheaters meet their match: Thank you, Richard Quinn! Retrieved from http://www.youtube.com/watch?v=7AdYAUe8q9w&feature=youtu.be

Zeichner, K. M., & Liston, D. P. (1996). *Reflective teaching: An introduction.* Mahwah, NJ: Lawrence Erlbaum Associates.

Zins, J. E., Weissberg, P. R., Wang, M. C., & Walberg, H. J. (Eds.). (2004). *Building academic success and social and emotional learning: What does the research say?* New York, NY: Teachers College Press.

Zweig, C. & Abrams, J. (1991). *Meeting the shadow: The hidden power of the dark side of human nature.* Los Angeles, CA: Jeremy P. Tarcher, Inc.

WEBSITES

America's Got Talent, music. http://youtu.be/pL2s2SWL8QE

Ayn Rand, Rationalism, 1970s. http://youtu.be/1ooKsv_SX4Y

Ayn Rand, Rationalism, 1980s. http://youtu.be/4doTzCs9lEc

Bill Cosby, *I don't know.* http://youtu.be/8ysFvUizRj8

Bill Cosby, *Creative learning.* http://www.youtube.com/watch?v=5-2NmLTdSq8

Bloom's Taxonomy, *Current uses.* http://www.nwlink.com/~donclark/hrd/bloom.html.

Bohr and Heisenberg's Theories, http://youtu.be/45KGS1Ro-sc

Brain Teasers. http://www.positscience.com/brain-resources/brain-teasers/scrambled-text

Carl Rogers, Humanist therapy. http://youtu.be/m30jsZx_Ngs

Confidence intervals. http://en.wikipedia.org/wiki/Confidence_interval

The Doctor, movie trailer. http://www.youtube.com/movie/the-doctor?feature=mv_sr

Dr. Jekyll and Mr. Hyde. http://youtu.be/aBxCUSUUbdc

Double Slit (Young) Experiments. http://en.wikipedia.org/wiki/Double-slit_experiment

Emoto's water studies. http://youtu.be/33IiYb8htHk

The Fight Club, movie trailer. movies.yahoo.com/movie/fight-club/trailers/

Fitz Perls, Gestalt therapy. http://youtu.be/T3jYcDbcpUs

Jacob Moreno, *Historical psychodrama.* http://youtu.be/zvgnOVfLn4k

Kevin Kern music. http://www.myspace.com/kevinkernmusic - !

The Kid, movie trailer. http://www.imdb.com/title/tt0219854/

Lave Wenger. http://www.learning-theories.com/communities-of-practice-lave-and-wenger.html

The Matrix, scene. http://youtu.be/wmYoN_pJ3RA

M. C. Escher. (2000). http://www.mcescher.com/Biography/biography.htm

Multiple Positioning, Entanglement, and the Young Experiments. http://youtu.be/v0v-cvvyc-M

North Korean guitarist. http://youtu.be/gSedE5sU3uc

PEAR, intention research center. http://www.princeton.edu/~pear/

Peter Gabriel, music. http://youtu.be/wkXeUE5gvRs

Portia Nelson. http://www.panhala.net/Archive/Autobiography.html

PowerPoint by Paradi. www.ThinkOutsideTheSlide.com

PowerPoint by Paradi. http://pptideas.blogspot.com/2012/07/presentation-tip-how-to-use-about-us.html

Presentation Etiquette. http://www.muchmorebi.com/powerpoint_etiquette.htm Yield Signs. http://www.trafficsign.us/yellowyield.html

Quantum Mechanics—What it means. http://youtu.be/7u_UQG1La1o

Simon & Garfunkel, Scarborough Fair. http://youtu.be/L-JQ1q-13Ek

Taylor Caldwell. http://www.goodreads.com/book/show/369088.The_Listener

Yoda in Star Wars. http://youtubecom/GITb6rzpTWM

Young Experiments. http://youtu.be/v0v-cvvyc-M and http://en.wikipedia.org/wiki/Double-slit_experiment.

Zerka Moreno, *Historical psychodrama*. http://youtu.be/VQUtxDK5V-w

Index